Why Can't I Drink Like *Everyone* Else?

One book can change your life forever. Rachel Hart has written that book. If you are someone who has struggled with drinking too much and struggled with finding a way to stop, look no further. When I was drinking too much, I would spend hungover mornings scouring the Internet and bookstores for a solution to drink less. I wanted to know how to do it, what to tell my friends, how to have a good night without it, and how to do all of that without attending one AA meeting. I couldn't find it.

Then came Rachel. Rachel literally changed my life with one sentence, "My life is way better without alcohol." I believed her. She was an intelligent, beautiful, successful and funny woman and she didn't drink. She wasn't in AA. She used to love alcohol and now she didn't. She wasn't just surviving a life without it; she was thriving.

I wanted to know how. I wanted every single detail. I wanted what she had. Fortunately for all of us, she has written this book telling us how exactly to do it. She doesn't just teach us what to do; she teaches us why. The why is what makes it easy to maintain. The why is what helps us stop beating ourselves up, stop using willpower, and ultimately stop suffering. It's the book that can hand you back your power to take a break from drinking, but more importantly, understand what it was all about in the first place.

She reminds us that drinking too much is not a character flaw. It's a learned habit. It makes sense that we do it. Ultimately, she shows us that we don't have to completely change who we are to stop drinking. In fact, we need to do the opposite. We just need to be willing to be with ourselves without the escape. It's a gentle and kind process, not one that insists our character flaws are the cause of our shortcomings. Drinking isn't a shortcoming; it's a misguided way to feel better. Our desire to feel better is good, not bad.

If you drink more than you want, I beg you to read this book immediately. Do everything she suggests. Hire her to help you. She was absolutely right; my life is so much better without alcohol. She's not just a perfect example of that being true, but also a very wise teacher and coach who can show you the way. I couldn't recommend her work more.

—**Brooke Castillo**, Master Coach Instructor and Founder of the Life Coach School

Rachel Hart is a wise and compassionate guide who offers an effective, evidence-based strategy for those looking for a way out of problem drinking. As someone who has "walked the talk," Rachel utilizes a combination of tools and insights to weave together a unique, jargon-free book that is filled with personal anecdotes, exercises, and insights that readers will find very useful and engaging. This book is already on my "recommended reading list" for my clients.

—**Phillip Cha**, LMFT

With a voice full of compassion, Rachel Hart takes the readers by the hand and offers to lead them on a step-by-step journey away from their despair about drinking.

—**Stephen Grimes**, LCSW, ACT

Why Can't
I Drink Like
Everyone
Else?

A STEP-BY-STEP GUIDE TO
UNDERSTANDING WHY
YOU DRINK AND KNOWING
HOW TO TAKE A BREAK

RACHEL HART

NEW YORK

NASHVILLE • MELBOURNE • VANCOUVER

Why Can't I Drink Like *Everyone* Else?
A STEP-BY-STEP GUIDE TO UNDERSTANDING WHY YOU DRINK AND KNOWING HOW TO TAKE A BREAK

Published in New York, New York, by Morgan James Publishing in partnership with Difference Press. Morgan James is a trademark of Morgan James, LLC. www.MorganJamesPublishing.com

The Morgan James Speakers Group can bring authors to your live event. For more information or to book an event visit The Morgan James Speakers Group at www.TheMorganJamesSpeakersGroup.com.

ISBN 978-1-68350-480-1 paperback
ISBN 978-1-68350-481-8 eBook
Library of Congress Control Number: 2017902787

Editing: Cynthia Kane

Author's photo courtesy of Hazel & Pine

Cover Design by:
Rachel Lopez
www.r2cdesign.com

Interior Design by:
Bonnie Bushman
The Whole Caboodle Graphic Design

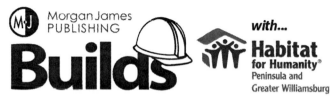

In an effort to support local communities, raise awareness and funds, Morgan James Publishing donates a percentage of all book sales for the life of each book to Habitat for Humanity Peninsula and Greater Williamsburg.

Get involved today! Visit
www.MorganJamesBuilds.com

Dedication

To everyone who offered their love and support.
You know who you are.

Table of Contents

Author's Note   *xiii*

Introduction   *xv*

1   My Story   1
2   A Different Perspective   14
3   The Role of Your Thoughts   35
4   The Role of Your Emotions   60
5   The Role of Your Urges   75
6   How to Take a Break from Drinking   96
7   Overcoming Common Obstacles   118
8   How to Feel Better   127
    Conclusion   136

Acknowledgements   *139*
About the Author   *141*
Thank You   *142*

Author's Note

As you read through this book, you'll notice that I don't use the labels alcoholic, addict, sober, or recovery to describe my story. Throughout college and my twenties, alcohol was a source of a lot of fun and a lot of problems in my life. During this period, I had an on-again, off-again relationship with drinking. For too long I struggled on my own because the only help and resources I could find required wearing a label for the rest of my life, and that didn't feel right.

I don't believe it makes sense to divide the world into "normal" drinkers and alcoholics. This black-and-white thinking leaves a lot of people who don't feel like they belong in either camp out in the cold. The way people use and interact with alcohol changes over time and in different contexts. Labels don't reflect these kinds of ebbs and flows or the different degrees of struggle.

Labels reduce a complex, multifaceted person into a single behavior. Some people find labels empowering. Other people find them stigmatizing, especially when a predominate cultural narrative connected to a specific label is rife with stigma, shame, and stereotypes. In my case, I don't identify as an alcoholic, sober, or recovered. These labels aren't useful for me or an accurate reflection of my journey. Ultimately, it's up to you to decide what feels right and go from there.

Addiction is real. This book is not for people who are addicted, non-functioning, or need medical attention.

Introduction

My brain had to be missing an off-switch. I don't remember when I decided this was the reason I took things too far when I drank, but it was the only plausible explanation I could come up with. Once I finished that first drink, I almost always wanted another. The signal inside of me that was supposed to tell me to "quit while I was ahead" didn't work properly.

Can you relate? If a little is good, more must be better. At least that's how it seems your brain is wired. Maybe you've even noticed that the desire to overdo things isn't unique to alcohol (for me, smoking really fast and eating too much, too quickly were right up there with guzzling a beer). Why is that? Why can't you be more like your best friend who knows when to call it a night? Why don't you drink like everyone else? You know you could stop drinking entirely—you don't *need* to drink— but why would you want to?

xvi | Why Can't I Drink Like *Everyone* Else?

Drinking is just what people do, and it's fun—*a lot* of fun. It's a recipe for a good time, a part of every celebration. After a couple of drinks, you can let your guard down, and the conversation flows. For a little while, you can forget about life and relax. With a little bit of a buzz going, you're not worried about what people think. You're not wrapped up in self-doubt. It's one of the few times you're not stuck in your head, overthinking everything. You're just enjoying yourself.

In college, getting drunk was a rite of passage. It gave you the permission you needed to be crazy and wild and even a little reckless. It dialed up your bravery. You didn't know what the night would bring and that was the whole point. You and your friends took turns taking care of each other when one of you took things too far. The next day, you would compare notes, nursing hangovers while you pieced together the night. This was a normal part of growing up and you were all for having your fun while you still could. Someday, you'd be old and boring and saddled with responsibilities, but thankfully you still had time.

As you grew up, so did your drinking. Red plastic cups turned into fine stemware and weighty tumblers. You compare cabernets to pinots. You don't just ask for gin, you request Hendricks. Sticky sweet concoctions gave way to master mixologists and cocktails named Death in Venice. Your drink selections are now a marker of who you are. Drinking is still fun, now it's also sophisticated. Plus it's a reliable break from always having to be so responsible all the time. Some days you can't wait to get home so you can pour yourself a glass and finally take the edge off.

Still, something doesn't feel quite right. Drinking has a pull on you that you don't understand and you don't like to acknowledge. That off-switch of yours, after all this time it's still unpredictable. Even though the way you drink has changed, you can still find yourself drinking more than you planned. Your tally of next-day regrets is growing. Everyone says and does stupid things when they're drunk. Everyone has nights they wish they could take back. But shouldn't you have grown out of this by now? Things that were funny in college now make you wince. Waking up with the same stupid repercussions over and over again has become tiresome.

Obviously, you've already tried to figure this out on your own. You've devised solutions to reign yourself in: deciding how many drinks you'll have before going out, only drinking on certain days, spacing out drinks or alternating with water, drinking only on a full stomach, drinking only certain types of liquor, or keeping pace with a friend who's less likely to go overboard. Sometimes they work. Other times it's a disaster.

Maybe you've heard that if you can't control how much you drink it's because you have a disease. You should admit that you're powerless over alcohol and attend meetings for the rest of your life. But even the thought of having to assume a label to explain your struggle makes you feel terrible and has you running in the opposite direction.

You want to change, but a life without alcohol looks miserable. What would you do while everyone else is out drinking? Who would you hang out with? What if you're still on the dating scene? How would you meet people? What if going out for drinks is the cornerstone of your social life? The last thing you want is to be the awkward person in the corner ordering club sodas from here on out. Maybe you've even quit before and your fears were confirmed. You appreciated waking up clear-headed, but nothing else about being sober was fun. You want to solve this problem, but you don't know how.

I know what it's like to feel stuck. I wrote this book because when I was struggling to understand why I drank the way I did, I couldn't find anything else like it. Everything I found required that I "admit" to being an alcoholic and wear a label for the rest of my life. I didn't want to sign up for a framework that said I was powerless or focused on "defects of character." If the 12-Steps work for you, keep doing what you're doing. But if they don't resonate, it doesn't mean you're in denial or not trying hard enough. There are seven billion people on this planet. The idea that a single solution exists for everyone never made sense to me. There's more than one way forward.

This book will teach you the tools the helped me, the same ones I use every day with my life coach clients. You won't ever hear from me that you *must* stop drinking, or that you'd really be better off if you did, or that cutting out alcohol will magically solve all your problems. The decision about whether you want to drink will always be yours and yours alone. Certainly, when I was torn about what to do, no amount of pleading or cajoling or harsh words could have persuaded me to change. I needed to decide what was right for me on my own.

What I will promise is this: it's possible to get to a place where drinking no longer has a pull over you and you won't feel like you're missing out. If you're rolling your eyes right now, I get it. When this was my struggle, I would have read a statement like that and told myself the person writing it was either crazy or fooling herself or both. But I probably would've also kept on reading, albeit skeptically, because I was frustrated that my drinking was still the source of so many of my problems. I was tired of waking up in the morning trying to piece together the previous night and worried about what I had said or done. I was embarrassed. I just wanted my drinking not to be an issue. More than anything, I wanted an answer to the question that plagued me: "Why can't I drink like everyone else?" This book will help you understand this question as it relates to you and show you how to shift your relationship with alcohol so that you can get to a healthier and happier place. Let's get started.

1 My Story

From Hang-ups to Hook-ups

I still remember my first college party. Well, that's not entirely true. I remember how it began. Days earlier I had arrived at my dream school. Wellesley, a women's college on the outskirts of Boston, has a long and storied reputation of producing women who shatter glass ceilings and make their mark on the world. It wasn't just my top-choice. It was the only college I applied to. I worked my butt off in high school to secure a spot, because more than anything else, I wanted to be one of those women.

In high school, I had no problem sitting in the front row of class or raising my hand. Academics were one thing; socializing was another. I was as outspoken in the classroom as I was uncomfortable socially. I bounced around friend groups, never quite fitting in. Standing in a darkened gymnasium during a school dance was excruciating.

The dichotomy between my behavior couldn't have been more stark: confident in one setting and a ball of insecurity in the other. While I didn't have much experience with partying or alcohol in high school, I had a lot of experience feeling out of place. College was my chance for things to be different.

Walking down Beacon Street in Boston toward that first party, I knew I was not off to a good start. My insides felt just as they had on car rides to high school dances—I couldn't tell if I needed to pass out or run to the bathroom. I had zero game plan for that party. Would there be alcohol? Would I drink? What would I do if someone offered? I just remember hoping that things would finally feel different. High school was over. I was in college now. Far away from the person I didn't want to be. My first days of college had gotten off to a good start, and I prayed that all my social hang-ups from high school wouldn't follow me. But walking toward that party felt like déjà vu.

Standing in the darkened room, I realized how wrong I had been. Distance hadn't changed me. I was still the same Rachel I had been in high school, and at that moment I wanted to disappear. Looking around, I didn't understand how everyone else appeared so at ease. My whole body was fighting the urge to run while my insides knotted tighter. Nothing about my body felt right. It was as if I was suddenly missing the instructions on how to stand or where to put my hands. I kept looking at the other women for cues about what I should be doing. Maybe I could slip away and take the bus back to campus and no one would notice? But then I found my solution.

I don't know what was in that punch, but it was sweet enough to mask the sting going down, and that was good enough for me. It wasn't even the buzz that felt good at first; it was the relief of having something to do with my hands. It may sound odd, but holding a drink gave my body a purpose. I felt awkward and exposed standing there; with a drink in my hand, I had a task. Something to hold. Something to drink. Something to refill. As my body figured out its purpose, the warm sensation, that started in my chest, moved to my head. With it, the scene before me transformed. I stopped searching for an escape route and started thinking that the party could be fun.

This wasn't my first experience drinking. In the months before college, I had tried alcohol on three occasions, but in much smaller settings. Each time with only a handful of people I already knew in spaces that felt more contained and where my anxiety wasn't in full swing. This time was different. I was a ball of nerves until suddenly I wasn't. If this was how alcohol made me feel, then sign me up.

Who knows how many times I filled up my cup that night, but soon enough my buzz turned into a full room tilt. I stumbled from one room to the next hunting for a place to sit down. The next thing I remember, one of the women I had come to the party with was shaking me awake, insisting that we had to catch the last bus home. Next to her, looking concerned, was a very tall, very handsome guy. Before I had time to be humiliated for passing out on a couch at my first college party, he had his arm around me and was helping me to my feet. Despite being wasted, part of me was still able to take in the scene: an extremely attractive man was, for some unknown reason, holding me close and *wanting* to walk me to the bus stop to make sure I got home okay. Months earlier, a guy like this wouldn't have given me the time of day. But that night the roles had reversed, and he seemed concerned. Things had changed.

Looking back on that early encounter with alcohol, I wonder if my belief that things had gone so well at that first college party contributed to how my drinking would go so wrong later on. I don't for a second wish that something bad had happened to me that night, because let's be honest, far too often on college campuses something does. But the lesson I learned at that party was one I would repeat over and over again during those four years and throughout my twenties. Feel uncomfortable, out of place, awkward: just drink as quickly as possible until the feeling goes away—even to the point of losing control. Alcohol became the perfect remedy to fix how I felt on the inside. The insecurity that gnawed at me before going out disappeared. The hang-ups whispering in my ear dissolved. Drinking became part and parcel of meeting guys. When I drank, the woman I wanted to be stepped forward: outgoing, fun, and sexy. During the week, I put my nose to the grindstone, but once the weekend rolled around I was ready to become the Rachel I wanted to be.

If I was worried about my behavior in college, I rarely let it show. I certainly wasn't going out and getting drunk on my own. Sure, I overdid it sometimes, but so did everyone else. I told myself that getting wasted every weekend was normal. Anyway, drinking was the only time I felt confident and attractive, and I saw absolutely no reason to mess with a good thing. Hangovers, while sometimes nasty, were still easy to shake off.

That's not to say I was completely oblivious to the downsides. At times, I worried that alcohol was turning into a crutch when it came to socializing. The more I needed it to feel at ease, the more I tended to go overboard. I also wasn't sure how I felt about the fact that all my romantic relationships seemed to start when I had one too many. Deep down, I wasn't always comfortable with my drunken antics, but I almost never let myself really dwell on these thoughts. My solution was to find a way to laugh about it and move on.

It wasn't until I moved to New York City after graduation that I had to face that something was not right with my drinking. Getting blackout drunk in the relative safety of my women's college was one thing. Getting blackout drunk in a city of eight-million people was another. Less than two months into my first real job, an after-work celebration with co-workers spiraled into being wasted, alone, and lost, in a city I barely knew. This wasn't stumbling around a picturesque college campus anymore; this was getting incapacitated in the real world. My memories are hazy at best, but despite making my way back to my neighborhood, I was so turned around and so intoxicated that all I could do was sit down on the curb to cry. I awoke, sometime later, having no idea how long I had been there and realizing I had passed out next to a car, alone, at night, on the streets of Manhattan.

Unharmed, but scared by my behavior, it suddenly seemed that the normal makings of countless crazy nights in college were actually reckless and stupid. I promised myself I would try to moderate, but I knew that wasn't really something I was good at. A few short weeks after my 22nd birthday, I decided it was time to stop altogether. This terrified me, but I made up my mind that enough was enough. I was sick of my behavior. I was tired of waking up and piecing together the previous night's events. The antics that I wrote off as the makings of a good story in college weren't so funny anymore. Something had to give.

The problem was I had no idea who I was without a glass in my hand. Sure, I knew who I was when it came to work: give me an assignment and a deadline and I would get it done, no problem. But socializing was another story. I felt like an enigma, even to myself. I was 17 at the first college party, and from that point forward alcohol was by my side whenever it came to having fun. Being underage barely mattered. There was always a way to get drunk. When I turned 21 during my senior year of college, it was only really notable because I could now go do in the open what I had done every weekend behind closed doors—get wasted. For me, alcohol was a crutch that I didn't know how not to need. The real me was hidden behind a blur of alcohol and I wanted to meet that woman.

When I summoned the courage to tell some of my close friends, they looked at me quizzically. (I didn't dare tell people until I had a month of not drinking under my belt—first and foremost I was terrified of failing.) Most people were cautiously supportive, but I always got the same question: how long would my enforced sobriety last? In retrospect, I think they didn't get it—everyone we knew drank a lot. But to be fair,

I was just as confused as they were. I didn't need alcohol to get through the day. I wasn't tippling from a secret flask. I drank socially. I drank at parties. I drank at bars. I drank a lot, but so did every twenty-something around me. Still, I was secretly worried that I kept taking things too far. Other people seemed to get to a point in the night when they called it quits. My off-switch didn't function properly. The attempts I made at moderating were hit and miss, and quitting seemed like the only way.

For an entire year, I stopped drinking. I must have turned down 1,000 drinks while I tried to navigate the social scene in New York. I went out. I went to parties. I went to bars. I even started dating someone. All without a drink in my hand. I woke up without hangovers. No longer lying in bed wondering what embarrassing things I had said or done the night before. Now that I didn't need to recover from a night of hard partying, I was insanely productive on the weekends.

Here's the part when I'm supposed to tell you that quitting was the best thing I ever did. That when I stopped drinking all my problems went away. Well, not exactly.

The problem was, I didn't particularly like the woman I discovered. She had so many flaws. So many things to fix. She was terrified of failing and obsessed with measuring up. She hated how she looked in the mirror and hated that she relied on attention from men to feel attractive. In a city as full of people as New York, she felt totally alone. Now that my life was in focus, all I could see was a litany of problems that I had no idea how to tackle. That entire year, I kept circling back to the same question: "If I'm this screwed up, why not just start drinking again?" Then at least I'd have a little relief.

On top of everything else, I was exhausted by being the odd-man out among friends. I was tired of having to constantly explain myself and answer people's questions about why I wasn't drinking. I was sick of rebuffing well-meaning friends who asked if I could make an exception, "just this once" because it was New Years, or someone's birthday, or they had purchased the most amazing bottle of wine. I kept turning them down, but inside I desperately wanted to go back to being like everyone else.

Finally, a year after I said no for the very first time, I didn't want to do it anymore. So I started drinking again, and I put almost no thought into it. A friend was visiting from out of town, and I decided I was sick of being different. I was sick of being the sober girl. I was sick of being a bore. I was sick of everything. Without saying a word, I marched into the kitchen of our shared apartment and grabbed a beer from the fridge, cracked it open, and gave myself some long-awaited relief from the tyranny of being me. Throughout my twenties, I would repeat this pattern over and over again. Flip flopping between periods of drinking and not drinking, all the while frustrated that I couldn't seem to make headway.

I just wanted to be a normal drinker, but as time wore on it seemed like my behavior stood out more and more. When my friends were still on their first glass, I was finishing up my second. I was usually the first one to flag down the waiter or head to the bar for another round. If a friend said she was done for the night, I tried to talk her into having one more. At the same time, drinking was everywhere and part of everything. I was convinced that unless I moved to a cabin in the woods, I could never avoid it. Plus, I had quit before and was miserable. I wasn't fun when I wasn't drinking. I felt stuck.

Whenever I hit a particularly low point, I would look for support. When I did, I usually ran into a bunch of walls. First, I was embarrassed to talk about my concerns. When I worked up the courage to broach the topic with close friends, I left the conversation feeling frustrated. Either I thought they didn't take me seriously, "Do you really think you have a problem?" or I was annoyed by advice, "Can't you just moderate? That's what I do." I knew people could change, because I watched friends who had partied alongside me in college become less interested in alcohol as time passed; but I didn't understand how that happened, and my own desire never seemed to abate. If they could change, why couldn't I?

Looking online wasn't much better. What I found was black and white. Either you were a normal drinker or you needed to fess up to being an alcoholic and the fact that you were powerless. To me, the 12-Steps looked like one big lesson in how I was screwed-up. I already knew all about my wrongs and short-comings and character defects. I had to live with them every day. A lifetime of attending meetings and introducing myself as "Hi, my name is Rachel and I'm an alcoholic" felt unbearable. I was in no man's land.

For a long time, I was convinced that my situation was different, unique. I was an outlier. I didn't understand why alcohol felt like a crutch that other people didn't seem to need. As much as I wanted someone to relate to what I was going through, I was sure no one could truly understand my situation. I was ashamed of my actions and ashamed I couldn't figure out a solution. I was unhappy when I drank too much and unhappy when I told myself I had to stop.

When I finally figured out a way forward that worked for me, it was as if the ground underneath me shifted. Alcohol was the source of many of my problems, yet the solution had very little to do with drinking. I finally understood why I used alcohol as a crutch and the reason letting go of it felt so impossible at times. Having a drink was a quick and easy fix when I felt awkward, insecure, and unhappy, and I had to figure out new ways to deal with these problems.

As I got more and more practice under my belt, it was unbelievable that I could no longer drink *and* feel like I wasn't missing out or constantly fighting off the desire to drink. In fact, the more I learned about what was driving my desire to drink, the more normal I felt. (This was a welcome break from always feeling there was something wrong with me.) The tools I will show you take consistent practice, but mastering them is so worthwhile.

All those years ago, when I arrived at Wellesley, I wanted to be a woman who tried to make a difference in the world. This book is certainly not what I imagined, but as a friend once pointed out to me, all those drunken nights and years of "wasted" time, were actually the best education I could've ever given myself. I hope what I've learned can help you too.

How Alcohol Becomes a Crutch

Alcohol was a crutch that I didn't know how not to need. It was a ticket out of social anxiety, a fail-safe way to put a lid on my internal-critic, and a recipe to meet guys. The idea of using alcohol as a crutch may resonate, but your experience may be entirely different. Why is that?

It's less about *how* you drink and more about *why* you drink. There are a million different things that people can use alcohol as a crutch for: stress, loneliness, boredom, anxiety, socializing, dating, difficult conversations, the holidays, insomnia, sex, insecurity, body shame, fear of failure, or even perfectionism. The common denominator is not the reason you turn to it, but what you learn when you do. That's right, *learn*. You teach yourself that alcohol solves a problem. The more you practice this lesson, the more ingrained it becomes. Alcohol doesn't become a crutch overnight. Like everything else you learn, it takes repetition.

Alcohol becomes a crutch when you unconsciously teach your brain that it makes a specific situation easier or a part of your life more bearable, usually because you don't have alternative means to cope with discomfort.

When my clients start working with me, they often describe a nagging sensation that something about their drinking doesn't feel quite right. Maybe they're concerned that they look forward to drinking a bit too much, or they hate waking up worried about what happened the night before. They might not like the physical repercussions—

headaches, grogginess, disturbed sleep, weight gain—or the emotional toll from beating themselves up after drinking more than they intended. They're often embarrassed to talk about this with anyone because they've been conditioned to believe that "normal" people don't ever struggle with their drinking. Their focus is all about *how* they are drinking, but focusing only on the how misses the big picture.

Here's an example. Sarah comes home to an empty apartment after work. This is her least favorite part of the day. Walking through the door is a reminder that she is all alone, and loneliness is not an emotion she likes to feel. At times, it's almost unbearable. Without even realizing it, she starts looking for a distraction. Pouring a glass of wine becomes a good temporary fix. It gives her a little buzz, and soon enough the weight of loneliness is no longer bearing down on her.

If Sarah does this once or twice, it's probably not a big deal. But what happens if this becomes her routine? What if it's the only way she knows how to deal with her loneliness, and so every evening she pours herself a glass of wine almost as soon as she kicks her shoes off? The more she repeats this behavior, the more her brain learns the following:

- There's something to look forward to at the end of the day. Once she walks through the door, there will be a hit of dopamine waiting for her as soon as she pours herself a drink, and
- Whenever loneliness bubbles up, she can find a little relief at the bottom of a glass.

Now keep in mind, Sarah's loneliness hasn't budged. She's just found a way to temporarily cover up how she's feeling. What she doesn't realize is that by repeatedly practicing this coping mechanism, she's creating a powerful habit in her brain. The longer these feelings go unaddressed, the more they will take root and the more she will feel drawn to pour herself another glass of wine to fix the situation.

At some point, Sarah might decide that she needs to cut back. Drinking in the evening is affecting her sleep. She's started waking up in the middle of the night, and in the morning she feels especially groggy. She might also be sick of her behavior. Thanks to her lowered inhibitions, she has a tendency to text her ex-boyfriend after a couple of glasses of wine. The next day, she feels embarrassed and regretful. Sarah wants to reign herself in, but now she has two problems to deal with:

- She has conditioned her brain to expect a reward at the end of the day. By the time 4pm rolls around, she's battling an intense urge to go home and open up a bottle of wine, and those urges are getting more and more difficult to resist.
- On the nights Sarah doesn't drink, she is by herself with her unbearable loneliness. The only way she knew how to deal with this feeling was by dulling it with a glass of wine, but without alcohol for a coping mechanism the nights she doesn't drink are miserable, and it's hard to stick to her resolve to cut back. At least a buzz made her feel temporarily better.

Unless Sarah understands how to handle her desire to drink while at the same time finding a different way to cope with feeling lonely, drinking is going to have a pull over her, and cutting back is going to feel challenging. Even if she does manage to temporarily stop drinking (which lots of people are able to do) she'll probably feel like she's missing out because having a drink was the one sure-fire way she had to feel better.

Most people don't understand the two pieces of this problem. When they can't immediately reign in their drinking or when cutting back feels difficult, they start to think that something might be wrong with them. Nothing is wrong. They've just unconsciously taught themselves a coping mechanism that brings with it a strong reward to keep using it. What they need to do is learn a new coping mechanism and how to handle their desire to drink, most people have no idea how to do this.

Alcohol changes our feeling state. When negative emotions arise, it's a quick and easy fix to temporarily dull the discomfort that accompanies them. The buzz you get from drinking is good at covering up how you're feeling, but it does nothing to eliminate what created the discomfort in the first place. If drinking becomes a regular coping mechanism to change how you feel, it usually brings with it a second set of problems— the repercussions of drinking too much. Ultimately, alcohol only disguises how you feel while the underlying problem continues to grow, and with it your desire to drink.

This explains why the year I stopped drinking in my early twenties was so miserable. Although I loved waking up clear-headed and not having to worry if I had done something embarrassing the night before, I missed the relief that drinking gave me so much that I eventually I started drinking again. Removing alcohol only fixed one set of problems—the ones created by drinking too much. I was able to resist the urge to drink over and over again, but I had no idea what to do about the social anxiety and the constant negative self-talk that barraged me. I couldn't shake the feeling that I was missing out because I had eliminated the only way I knew how to give myself relief.

I didn't realize that I needed to find a way to deal with the underlying problems that made alcohol so appealing in the first place. Until I figured out new ways to feel confident and at ease socially, alcohol would continue to have a pull over me. Once I learned how to solve these problems without drinking (using the tools I'll show you in the following chapters), my desire for alcohol slowly dissipated.

It's the difference between **problem-solving** and **problem-stalling**. Alcohol is a problem-staller. Your attention is temporarily diverted away from whatever discomfort you're feeling, but in the long-run alcohol does nothing to solve the underlying issues. All it does is temporarily mask them. Ultimately, there are two sets of problems at play:

- The underlying negative emotions that make the escape that alcohol gives you so appealing in the first place, or what I call your **underlying problems**, and
- The negative results from drinking too much, or as I call them your **aftermath problems**.

Removing alcohol from your life will certainly solve the repercussions from over-drinking. It won't do anything to change the negative emotions that alcohol was helping you escape from in the first place. (More on the distinction between underlying and aftermath problems and why you need to understand the difference in the next chapter.)

This is where the tools I'm going to teach you come in. By understanding new ways to solve the problems that alcohol is so good at covering up, you can start taking concrete steps that help you feel better and manage whatever is going on in your life. It's the difference between managing how you feel from the inside out and trying to feel better from the outside in.

2   A Different Perspective

Frameworks for Understanding Over-Drinking

Not being able to control my drinking made me feel broken. The more I struggled to understand what exactly was wrong with me, the more I became convinced that something inside just wasn't right, as if I had a fundamental flaw that corrupted my whole being.

Maybe you feel the same way? That the only explanation for drinking more than you intend, and making the same mistake over and over despite knowing full well the consequences, is that something must be wrong with you. A defect in the system. So many people who struggle with their drinking can relate. I find that many people, even those who back in the day I would've considered to be light drinkers, are ashamed to admit that they feel a pull toward drinking that they don't understand and can't always control. Even these people at times worry that this pull might mean something is wrong with them. Why is it that we've all come to the same conclusion?

You don't need to look further than at the most common frameworks for how we talk about people who struggle with alcohol:

- **People who drink too much have a disease.** It's not their fault; they're just sick. They have an illness that makes it so their brain doesn't properly function. Unlike normal people, their brain can't handle alcohol. It renders them powerless. The only cure is to remove the substance entirely.

- **People who drink too much have a character defect.** They prioritize pleasure over everything else, including their well-being and the well-being of their loved ones. They're selfish, master manipulators, and liars. The way out is to acknowledge their defects of character and atone for their wrongs and misdeeds. They must work at being a better person.

These models overlap, creating a foundation for most people to understand this problem. Is it any surprise that people who struggle with how much they drink often feel ashamed, or that even people who only occasionally feel as if they are pulled to drink more than what they intended are reluctant to tell anyone because it might mean they have to step into one or both of these boxes?

During my twenties, I felt trapped. These explanations didn't sit right with me, yet they were all that I knew. I rejected these explanations while simultaneously adopting some of these beliefs. How's that for confusing?

I was sure that something was wrong with me. My brain was missing something other people had. This made perfect sense because I could clearly see that some of my friends, even those who had partied alongside me in college, were better at knowing when to call it a night. I even watched as some of them seemed to magically grow out of their sloppy behavior. Similarly, although most of what I knew about 12-Steps wasn't appealing, I felt strongly that I needed to double down on being a better person. After all, my actions often left me feeling profoundly ashamed and embarrassed. A good person wouldn't act like that.

In retrospect, I think I rejected these frameworks because both signaled that something was wrong with me and I already felt plenty broken. Either I was signing up for there to be a something wrong with my brain (the **disease model**) or something wrong with who I was (the **character defect model**). Neither gave me the chance to be unbroken— the one thing I wanted more than anything else.

I felt broken long before I took my first drink. My very first school portrait is a vivid reminder of this. I was four years old and had just started kindergarten. The photographer tried to coax a smile out of me, but I wouldn't budge. I was only four, but I had already hated the large gap between my front teeth and I wasn't about to let him ruin my first school portrait by revealing my goofy grin. It's hard to look at the picture and see the beginnings of a little girl who had already learned to hate her appearance.

The feeling that something was wrong with me persisted throughout grade school. Through glasses and hearing problems and speech therapy, through remedial reading classes and the threat of being held back, it was always there. Friendships didn't come easily, and my over-eager attempts to fit in and make friends always seemed to miss the mark.

So no, I didn't feel broken *because* I struggled with my drinking. I felt this way years before I ever got drunk, and I was reluctant to seek out help that solidified what I already knew about myself: something was wrong with me.

It wasn't until my thirties that I learned that a third model existed that explained why I drank too much and didn't make me feel broken. In this model, over-drinking isn't a disease or a defect of character; rather, it is a coping mechanism that I unconsciously taught my brain:

- **People who drink too much taught themselves a habit that they can unlearn.** They unconsciously taught their brain to use alcohol as a coping mechanism to deal with negative emotions. Without information on how habits work or how to unravel them, efforts to change can be frustrating.

This definition resonated with my experience. I kept turning to alcohol, even as my regrets and misgivings mounted, because I didn't understand the habit I had created and didn't know another way forward in the face of discomfort. Instinctively, I already had some sense of this when I described alcohol as a crutch I didn't know how not to need. Almost as soon as I started drinking I understood that alcohol got rid of uncomfortable feelings, but I never realized that by repeating this technique over and over again I was teaching my brain to desire alcohol in certain situations.

This perspective gave me hope. If I had taught myself how to drink too much, maybe I could also teach myself how to stop? Not only that, maybe there wasn't anything wrong with my brain or my character? Perhaps I could work at changing the habits that no longer served me without signing up for more brokenness?

I knew I had one thing going for me: remember the girl who sat in the front row of class and wasn't afraid to raise her hand? If there was one thing I was confident in, it was my ability to learn. I didn't think I was the smartest person around, but I knew that I was studious. (By the way, your ability to learn a new way forward has nothing to do with how you did in school or your grade point average. Learning is what every brain is designed to do. You're learning all the time, whether you know it or not. Just because changing a habit can be hard at first doesn't mean anything is wrong.)

Not only that, but the learning model also meant that the idea of life-long treatment (e.g., attending meetings for the rest of my life) or assuming a label (Hi, my name is Rachel and I'm an alcoholic) wasn't necessary. My struggle with drinking didn't have to become an identity that I wore or a reflection of who I was as a person. It was just a habit I needed to unlearn.

At this point, most people have the same question: aren't some people predisposed to struggle with addictive behaviors? There's no doubt that genetic predispositions and environmental factors can play a role, but your genes, your socioeconomic status, and your past, are not your destiny. For most people, this comes as a relief. You're not doomed to struggle, and the world is not divided into "normal" drinkers and alcoholics. This dichotomy ignores the many different degrees of struggle and the fact that people's drinking can change over time and under different circumstances.

I'm grateful that I eventually found a group of people who talked about over-drinking in a different way. I was first introduced to some of these concepts through a group called SMART Recovery, a peer-support group that uses techniques from cognitive behavior therapy to help people understand and control their use of drugs and alcohol. It took me months to finally walk through the door of my first group meeting on the Upper East Side of Manhattan. But once the meeting began, I started to relax. No one was telling me that I had a disease or that I needed to call myself an alcoholic (in fact, SMART discourages the use of labels like alcoholic and addict). I wasn't there to confess all the bad things I had ever done while drunk, admit the nature of my wrongs, or ask for a higher power to remove my defects of character or shortcomings. All I had to do was start learning and applying new tools.

The Think → Feel → Act Cycle

The tools I first learned opened my eyes to a simple, yet radical cycle: think → feel → act. In other words, the things you do (i.e., your actions, including drinking) don't just spontaneously happen. They're driven by how you feel. Your feelings (or emotions) also don't appear out of the blue. They're generated by your thoughts. The cycle works like this: you think a thought, which creates a feeling, which propels you to act. Think → feel → act. It's about as simple as it gets.

This concept isn't new. You can trace its roots all the way back to ancient Greece. Philosophers like Epictetus put it this way:

> *"Men are disturbed **not** by the things that happen,*
> *but by their **opinion** of the things that happen."*

In short, if you want to understand *why* you feel the way you do, you don't need to search your environment. Your feelings aren't caused by what's happening to you; they're the result of what you *think* about what's happening to you. In other words, you never feel an emotion without first having a thought. The way you feel (i.e., your emotions) is the result of a thought. If you want to understand why you feel the way you do, you only need to look inside your mind and examine your thinking.

The **think** → **feel** → **act** cycle explains why no two people react the same way to identical events. The way an individual feels about the events in her life is a result of what she thinks about those events. Take the weather. A rainy day doesn't cause your emotions. Before you have an emotion, you always think a thought. The person who looks outside and thinks "This rain is going to ruin my commute" will probably feel annoyed. Whereas someone else who sees the same weather outside and thinks "My garden is going to love this rain" will probably feel grateful. The rain doesn't create their emotions; their thoughts about the rain do. Most of us believe differently and think the cycle works like this: **life happens → feel → act**. We attribute how we feel to everything happening to us, and don't understand the role of our thoughts.

Of course, when I started this work, I was more interested in changing my actions, i.e., how much I was drinking. Understanding that my thoughts created my feelings was fine, but I wanted to know why curbing my drinking was so challenging. Here again, this framework provides clues: if emotions drive your actions, then **if you want to understand why you do what you do, you needed to look no further than how you feel**.

This concept is especially interesting if you're using alcohol as a crutch to escape feeling uncomfortable. I was always running from my negative emotions because I thought I had no other choice—I thought feeling better meant changing what was happening in my life. It's why so many of us focus on our job, our bank account, our bodies, our relationship status, etc. as the key to happiness. We think that our external environment creates how we feel and ignore the role of our thoughts. The think → feel → act cycle provides a different way forward. How you think is the key to changing how you feel and how you act. If you're using alcohol as a crutch, being able to change both areas is crucial.

The think → feel → act cycle is also why I believe it's possible to get to a place where you don't desire to drink. If alcohol is the thing creating your desire, then you're stuck. Because alcohol isn't going anywhere. It's been with us for thousands of years and is going to stay. On the other hand, if your thoughts create your desire, you're in luck. From this position, you can observe, change, practice, and eventually develop new automatic thoughts associated with drinking.

Repetition and Habits

Think → feel → act. This cycle is always working in the background of your brain. The more you repeat certain thoughts or actions, the more you solidify specific patterns. Sometimes we do this consciously (e.g., learning to drive a car), but lots of us hardwire habits into our brains unconsciously (e.g., using alcohol as a crutch). The good news is that your brain is built to run on habits; you just need to learn how to harness them.

People learn through repetition. You repeat something until your brain becomes so good at it that the steps become unconscious. Indeed, being able to do things without thinking is what makes humans so efficient. Take driving a car. How exhausting would it be if every time you got behind the wheel you had to concentrate on the hundreds of steps involved in driving? It takes practice, but after a while most people can just get into the car and go—the individual steps of driving no longer cross our mind. The habit is so hardwired into our unconscious that we can execute the hundreds of steps involved in driving and find our mind wandering at the same time. The habit is so ingrained that our brain is free to do other things.

Habits save your brain energy, and more than anything your brain wants to be efficient. The unconscious nature of habits is both extremely useful and—when you want to change a habit like over-drinking—extremely frustrating. This is largely because few of us understand how the think → feel → act cycle works and the role it plays in creating habits. Without understanding this process, we find ourselves trying to undo a habit without understanding how it works.

When you're stuck in a negative habit, like over-drinking, you don't have the first clue how to begin to change it (other than using willpower, which most people find doesn't last). It's no wonder then that the disease model ("I can't help it; I was born this way") or the character defect model ("I can fix this by being a better person") are at times appealing. We don't understand why change feels so difficult, and it's easy to believe that our struggle is a sign that something is wrong with us. These models offer explanations for a problem that is baffling precisely because it is unconscious. Unfortunately, for many people these models can reinforce shame-producing thoughts (e.g., "Something is wrong with me."). Of all your emotions, shame is not very motivating. You're more likely to feel so bad that you want to give up and believe that change is impossible.

The Learning Model

At times, I felt like I was drinking against my will. I knew I shouldn't have that fourth glass of wine, but even though I had made a plan before the night began it was usually no match for the habit I had taught myself. Largely because I had no idea what was driving my habit to over-drink. Once I understood the think → feel → act cycle and how it applies to drinking, it finally made sense why when I had a lot of negative thoughts (and by extension a lot of negative emotions), it was much harder to control how much I drank. All I wanted to do was not feel what I was feeling, and my brain had already learned the perfect solution—dull the way I felt with alcohol. At the time, I didn't understand what was going on or that I had actually taught my brain this coping mechanism.

The learning model fascinated me because it applied to all habits—not just drinking. Indeed, the tools I will walk you through in this book are not unique to drinking, but are useful in many different contexts. Outside of the realm of alcohol and drugs, almost everyone agrees that habits are difficult to change. If you've ever tried to lose weight, stick to an exercise plan, or save money, you know how hard it can be to break the bad habits that compel you to mindlessly eat a bag of chips, hit the snooze button instead of going for a run, or stick to a budget. However, when it comes to alcohol, most of us believe that we should just be able to change how much we drink without any struggle.

It takes effort to break old habits and replace them with new ones. When you struggle or have a setback, it doesn't mean there's anything wrong with your brain or that you just need to work at being a better person. It just means that your brain is learning something new. Just like the very first time you got behind the wheel of a car. You didn't master driving on your first attempt, nor will you learn a new habit right out of the gate. It takes repetition and practice to replace a habit like over-drinking with something new, but it's most certainly possible. The key is to use the **think** → **feel** → **act** cycle to learn what is driving the habit and harness the cycle to change it.

What You Learn from Drinking

Remember how I said that I wondered if my early encounter with alcohol in college contributed to how drinking became a problem for me later? Yes, I definitely got way too drunk, way too quickly that night. But there are two important pieces to understand.

Long before I ever started over-drinking, I had a habit of eating really quickly to the point that I made myself physically uncomfortable. Around seventh or eighth grade, I would come home to an empty house after school. Every afternoon I would fix myself a snack, and then another, and another until the only thing I could feel was being uncomfortably full. I struggled as a teenager, and overeating to the point of zoning out was the only way I knew how to escape how I felt inside. Essentially, I was using food to divert energy away from my brain and my nervous system (where my negative self-talk was in high-gear) and direct it toward my digestive system. By giving my body a surplus of food to contend with, I was actually able to dull how I was feeling. No one taught me how to do this. All by myself I found a way to numb myself and made a habit of it, long before alcohol ever entered the picture.

When the feelings of anxiety knotted in my stomach at the party, I couldn't make the feeling go away with food. It's probably why my first thought was to escape. But before I did, I had a drink and noticed that the feeling started to lessen. Was I conscious of this? Not entirely. I just knew that one moment I felt like crawling out of my skin and then suddenly I started feeling better.

So why did I overdo it that night? I suppose there could be lots of reasons, but I think my lonely and unhappy afternoons of my childhood contain a clue. My preferred method for distracting myself from an uncomfortable feeling was turning to an outside substance and consuming it as quickly as possible—going back for more and more—until the emotional discomfort lessened. Obviously, the repercussions from over-drinking were more significant for me than the repercussions from over-eating, but the pattern of numbing an uncomfortable emotion by overdoing it on an outside substance was well-established long before I showed up at college.

The second piece to understand is what I learned afterwards. When I woke up the next day, I was at first embarrassed. But no one really treated what had happened as a big deal. It was funny. We all laughed about it. And the tall, handsome stranger who had helped me to the bus? He ended up contacting me to see how I was. My 17-year-old brain viewed this as a good thing. I escaped feeling awkward, I had fun, and I met a guy. What more could you ask for? In fact, weren't those the very things I hoped would happen? The next weekend, when my friends and I went out, it seemed only normal to repeat again what had already proved to work: get drunk, have fun. I repeated this pattern over and over again in college, until having fun, feeling confident, and hooking up all corresponded with drinking.

The learning model could offer clues for why my friends who partied just as hard as I did, might have had an easier time cutting back on how much they drank. They weren't necessarily learning the same thing from drinking as I was, because we weren't drinking for the same reasons. On the surface, it seemed like all of us were doing the same thing: going out, getting drunk, and having a good time. But I was drinking to get rid of my discomfort and teaching myself a coping mechanism I didn't yet fully understand. Getting drunk may not have had anything to do with ridding themselves of uncomfortable emotions.

I walked into those college parties with a ton of baggage. Remember the merciless self-critic who felt completely out of my element in social situations and my fixation on being perfect? I had no idea how to handle these problems, but as it turned out drinking solved all of them. It quieted my self-critic, put me at ease in social situations, and allowed me to let loose and step outside of the perfectionist box I had built for myself. It was the only way I knew how not to care what other people thought—at least as long as I was drunk.

Learning this coping mechanism at 17 is probably why the habit took hold relatively quickly. Before the age of 25, your brain hasn't fully finished developing, so habits take root more quickly. It's the same reason why learning a language is easier when you're younger. Your brain is still developing and is more plastic. Even though I got drunk at that very first party, my reliance on alcohol in social settings didn't just appear; it was something that unfolded over the course of many years as I kept practicing going to parties, getting drunk, feeling like I was finally free of myself, and getting the attention from guys that I so craved.

If it feels like suddenly you woke up to your drinking being a problem (which is how I felt at age 22), I bet your habit didn't appear overnight. It unfolded through a process of repetition. Because everyone is different, what you learn influences whether you want to repeat the behavior. As I said before, genetics and environmental influences can certainly play a role, but what you're learning is also crucial. It makes a lot of sense that different people learn different things when engaging in the same behavior. Someone who gets drunk and wakes up the next day thinking, "I never want to do that again. I hate the feeling of being out of control," has learned something different from someone like me who thinks, "Holy crap, this is how you stop feeling so awkward and insecure all the time?" Each person's think → feel → act cycle is unique. In other words, the relationship between the person and her individual response to drinking—including what she learns—matters a lot.

Where does this leave you? Whether you know it or not, your brain is learning something when you drink. Yes, alcohol gives you a hit of dopamine and a buzz, but that's not the only thing happening. You might also learn that alcohol is a quick and easy fix for dulling a negative emotion you don't want to feel. If you repeat this over and over again whenever a negative emotion arises, you may unknowingly create a habit of turning to alcohol to dull how you feel without ever realizing it. Without other ways of coping, alcohol develops a pull over you as a tried and true way to change how you feel.

Thankfully, you have the **think → feel → act** cycle to start to understand this. Your actions don't materialize out of thin air. There's always an emotion driving your actions and a thought that creates your emotion. When you feel like you're pulled to drink and don't understand why you drink despite knowing the consequences, it's helpful to understand the think → feel → act cycle working in the background that prompts you to pour yourself a drink in the first place. Identifying the cycle, and then ultimately learning how to influence and change it, is the key to changing what isn't serving you.

The Myth of the Normal Drinker

For years, I had one wish: to become a "normal" drinker. This was the obvious solution to my problems. That way I could still go out and have fun and avoid all the repercussions. Drinking too much was the problem. Drinking normally was the way out.

If you've ever worried about your drinking, then some version of this thought has probably crossed your mind. It's why you've probably spent time already trying to moderate before picking up this book. You could probably write a list of all the different things you've tried. Wanting to be a "normal" drinker creates a singular focus on moderation and a willingness to try almost anything to reach that goal.

Have you ever really thought about what exactly makes for a "normal" drinker? I used to toss around that term as if it was just an obvious distinction that everyone understood. So obvious, in fact, that I couldn't conceive of needing to define it. But it's worth spending some time considering what "normal" means to you, because my definition and your definition are in all likelihood unique to ourselves. Does this person never get drunk or is it that when she gets drunk she never does something she regrets? Is this person satisfied sipping a single glass of wine all night, or does she have a perfect understanding of where her limit is and never goes past it? Does she not desire alcohol or is she able resist the pull of wanting more? Does your "normal" drinker possess incredible tolerance or unwavering control?

It's important, to know what "normal" means to you because it will give you clues about how exactly drinking helps you. Because here's the thing: your drinking *does* help you. If there weren't any benefits, you wouldn't feel like giving up drinking meant a lifetime of missing out.

If your "normal" is being satisfied with a single glass of wine, and my "normal" is getting drunk but never blacking out, you and I are talking about two very different normals. The point is, there's no right answer. You just need to understand what normal means to you.

After quitting drinking for a year at 22, I was even more convinced that figuring out how to drink "normally" was the right approach. I was tired of being the odd-one out and answering everyone's questions about why I wasn't drinking anymore. I told myself that I wanted to fit in again. I wanted to be like everyone else. Figuring out how to drink normally would solve all of that.

In reality, I had a deeper motivation than just "fitting in." The year that I stopped, I saw who I was without a drink at my hand, and honestly I didn't really like her. She wasn't that much fun. In fact, she was kind of a head case. All my insecurities and hang-ups were on display. Everywhere I looked, I felt as if I wasn't measuring up. Without alcohol in my life, I no longer had relief from me. I didn't have a way to forget about all my problems and just have fun.

When I wasn't drinking, I was face-to-face with every problem that made drinking so appealing in the first place, and I had no idea what to do about it. Without a buzz, I was at the mercy of the constant chatter in my mind, chatter that amped up when I was in social situations. All I wanted was for my Friday nights to go back to being an excuse to cut loose and stop hating myself. Removing alcohol took away the option of slipping into the skin of a woman who was brave and bold and didn't care what people thought of her—if only for a night. I missed the respite from being me.

Don't get me wrong, drinking had real downsides, and stopping had real benefits. Chief among them was no longer spending the next day beating myself up for overdoing it and getting drunk. Despite not having to worry about hangovers or being embarrassed about my behavior, I missed "fun Rachel." I longed for the break from my life that was waiting for me at the bottom of a glass.

What I didn't know was that by focusing on being a "normal" drinker I was ignoring the complete picture of why I drank. Without this information, both drinking and not drinking would, and did, feel like a struggle.

It's the difference between what I introduced in Chapter 1: "underlying" and "aftermath" problems.

- **Aftermath problems** are the negative results of over-drinking; the consequences of drinking too much.

Hangovers and regretting what you did or said are all aftermath problems. Interestingly, these problems don't require that you drink a lot. If having two glasses of wine makes you more apt to pick a fight with your partner, that still counts. If you're experiencing a negative consequence it doesn't matter how much you had to drink. Aftermath problems are also the reason why being a "normal" drinker is so appealing. The "normal" drinker you imagine doesn't ever have these sorts of problems.

- **Underlying problems** are most often the negative emotions that you want to dull and that make drinking so appealing in the first place.

Underlying problems are there long before you ever picked up a glass and are almost always connected to your emotional state. Drinking is appealing because alcohol numbs, dulls, and distracts you from your underlying problems. Alcohol gives you a little bit of escape from the discomfort of how you feel.

When I was 22, quitting drinking resolved all the consequences from drinking too much. But it also left me helpless against the underlying problems that contributed to my desire to drink. I was using alcohol to get ride of feeling insecure, anxious, and awkward and had no idea how to deal with these problems on my own:

- **I was a merciless self-critic.** At the time, I didn't even understand that I was overly critical of myself. When I listed everything that was wrong with me, I thought I was just stating the truth, and the truth was I didn't measure up.
- **I felt completely out of my element in social situations, especially those that involved men.** Remember that feeling I described in my stomach in the previous chapter—not knowing

if I needed to pass out or run to the bathroom? I had no idea how to coexist with this feeling. I just wanted out.

- **I was fixated on doing everything perfectly.** I had zero coping mechanisms in place for when I failed to meet my impossible standards or to give myself a break when I was suffocating under the weight of so much pressure.

My brain discovered early on that alcohol gave me a respite from all three—at least as long as I was buzzed. Drinking quieted my self-critic. It put me at ease in social situations. It allowed me to blow off steam when I was stressed out, and it gave me permission to throw caution to the wind and be spontaneous. For an insecure perfectionist, drinking was a welcome break.

At the time, I didn't fully understand this. I thought drinking was fun and made meeting guys easier. I didn't understand how I had come to rely on alcohol to solve so many of my underlying problems. And the longer I used alcohol to distract myself from what was really going on, the more these problems grew and the tighter their grip was.

Now your underlying problems don't need to have been with you since childhood. They don't need to be traumatizing or even all that serious. They just need to be present *before* you take a drink and less bothersome once you have some level of alcohol in your system. Many of my clients describe it as the sensation of wanting to take the edge off at the end of the day. Whatever your edge is—whether it's stress about your job or anxiety about money or the loneliness you feel when you go home to an empty house—that's your underlying problem.

If you've contemplated changing how you drink, I bet your focus has been on reigning in the repercussions—the aftermath problems. For me, these were things like blacking-out, regrettable hook-ups, hangovers, and wanting to hide from the world because I was humiliated by my behavior. Remember, there's no litmus test for what counts as an aftermath problem—no level of severity that you must meet. Your aftermath problems are whatever negative results arise from your drinking, and they can appear if you drink a lot or a little.

When you're trying to get out from under a problem, focusing on the negative outcomes seems like the obvious place to start. It's why I thought being a "normal" drinker was the solution. If I could reign in all the consequences from over-drinking, I should be golden, right? In my mind, normal drinkers didn't black-out. Normal drinkers didn't spend the day trying to forget what they did last night. Normal drinkers could get a little crazy, but they only ever had fun. Being a "normal" drinker should fix all of this.

I thought the way to change was to just keep reminding myself how terrible I felt after a night of heavy drinking. If I remembered all the repercussions my drinking created, surely I would drink more responsibly. But I was ignoring the underlying problems—the very reason why drinking was so appealing in the first place.

Instead of asking, "How can I become a normal drinker?" I really should have been asking, "How does drinking help me?" It's the question that changes your focus from aftermath problems to underlying problems.

If you feel yourself not wanting to answer this question, don't worry. That's what happened to me at first and often happens to my clients. Looking at how drinking helped me felt like I was trying to fake a silver lining on a part of my life that was causing me pain. My resistance was so strong that it took me a long time to even consider that drinking may be helping me.

Answering this question can be the beginning of a huge shift in your life. Instead of fixating on the problems your drinking is causing, you can start understanding the problems it is solving. Shifting from your aftermath problems to the underlying problems can show you a new way forward.

Once I made this shift, my drinking started to make a lot of sense. I spent so much time beating myself up for repeating the same mistakes. I saw the failure to "learn my lesson" as proof that something was wrong with me. Looking at how drinking helped me felt productive. If I could learn new ways to solve my underlying problems, then maybe drinking would stop having the same pull over me. In fact, the more I learned that I didn't need alcohol to solve these problems, the less I desired it.

This is what the following chapters will teach you how to do. Learning these tools is the key to moving to a place where you can unravel you desire to drink.

Exercise 1: How Does Drinking Help You?

Time Required: 30 minutes—1 hour

The goal of this exercise is to shift your focus from your aftermath problems to your underlying problems. In short, you want to understand how drinking is helping you. Instead of fixating on the problems your drinking is causing, you can start understanding the problems it is solving. Your answers can show you a new way forward. You don't need to devote all your energy to becoming a "normal" drinker; you can think about what makes alcohol so appealing in the first place.

This exercise will let you consider how drinking is helping you. Set aside at least 30 minutes to read through and answer the questions. Take your time. Don't attempt to answer the questions in your head. Write them down. You'll want to refer back to your answers later.

Do your best to stay curious. If you start feeling uncomfortable or anxious, pause and take a deep breath. The information you're gathering is just that—information. What you write down is neither good nor bad. There are no right or wrong answers. Try to think of your responses as data points. The more data points you have, the better you can assess where you want to go from here.

The best place to start is looking at how and why you use alcohol and see if you can begin to identify any patterns. The following questions should give you more insight into the benefits associated with drinking:

- **When do you usually drink and why?** Think about when you usually drink and what you associate with that time. For example, coming home from work and fixing a drink signals that the day is over. Sharing a bottle of wine over dinner with your partner helps you open up and relax. Going out with friends on the weekend to celebrate the end of the work week.
- **What specifically do you like about drinking?** The taste, the smell, the social-aspect, the buzz? Be as specific as possible.
- **What situations does it improve or make easier?** Dating, spending time with your extended family, networking events, flying, insomnia, time alone, etc.?
- **How does it make these situations easier?** Be as specific as possible for how drinking helps in the moment.
- **List any specific emotions it helps with.** Anxiety, stress, boredom, loneliness, etc.?
- **How does alcohol help you deal with these emotions?** Does it numb you, help you escape, help you loosen up, make you more talkative, help you feel more confident, etc.?

Review your answers. Have you covered all the benefits? If not, add them in. Now that you've reviewed all the benefits, it's time to get really specific about the underlying problems alcohol helps you cope with. Remember, there is no litmus test for what qualifies as underlying problem: it just needs to be present *before* you take a drink and less bothersome once you have some level of alcohol in your system. Think of it this way, if alcohol helps you "take the edge off" your underlying problem is whatever that "edge" is for you. With your earlier responses in mind, answer the following questions:

- How does alcohol help you?
- What problem(s) is drinking solving for you?

As you work your way through this book, you'll want to keep these specific benefits in mind. The tools you will learn later will help you identify alternative means to solve these problems without alcohol. This is what focusing on the benefits is all about.

If you're skeptical of this approach, trust me. I get it. But ask yourself this: has it worked to focus on the downsides, what you're doing wrong, or beating yourself up? With shame at the helm, resolve never lasts long. Looking at the benefits is the beginning of trying a new way forward.

3 The Role of Your Thoughts

The Reason Willpower Is a Slog

Many of my clients tell me they just need to be more disciplined when it comes to drinking. For a long time I also believed willpower was the ticket to salvation. If I could just be more disciplined when it came to alcohol, I would solve my problem with over-drinking.

Here's the deal: willpower can certainly work, but most people find it feels like a slog. When I stopped drinking shortly after I turned 22, it was a long, drawn out battle with willpower. And it worked for a year. But all my energy and focus was on saying no. Turning down drinks at a party. Avoiding cocktails at happy hour. Declining wine with dinner. Saying no to a champagne toast at New Years. I said no over and over, and it wore on me because I still *really* wanted to drink. (If you've heard the term white-knuckling, this is what it looks like.) I didn't want to be different from my friends. I just wanted to be normal, and saying no a thousand times did not make me feel normal. Plus, it was exhausting.

There's an ongoing debate in the scientific community about willpower: do humans have a finite amount that decreases with use, or is your capacity for willpower determined by your personal beliefs about willpower itself (e.g., whether you *believe* you have a lot of willpower or very little of it)? Either way, willpower isn't a great strategy for long-term change because it focuses on the moment before you say yes to an action (in this case having a drink) rather than on what triggered your desire to act in the first place.

Here's where the **think** → **feel** → **act** cycle comes in. You exert willpower between the steps *feel* and *act*. The feeling that compels you to act is the desire to drink. You use willpower to resist this feeling. You use your will to say no to the action that your desire is driving (in this case, having a drink). The beauty of the think → feel → act cycle is that with practice you can intervene before your desire has been ignited. You do this by identifying the thought that is fueling your desire and working to change it. By harnessing the think → feel → act cycle, you can start to unwind your desire without needing to depend solely on willpower (this by the way is the long-game, and happens only with repeated practice).

When my willpower failed and I gave in to my desire to drink, I always saw it as a sign that I wasn't trying hard enough. If I just tried harder, if only I had more resolve, I should be able to stick to my commitment. I thought I was lazy, weak-willed and that everything would be better if I just tried harder. You might feel this way too. I know you might not be ready to give up on the idea that discipline is the answer, because you've been told over and over that willpower is the only way to undo a habit. But there is a more effective tactic. Either way, it doesn't make a whole lot of sense to wage war against a habit you unconsciously created when you don't fully understand what's driving it.

When I was 22, my only focus was on stopping the action: don't have a drink. I acted as if my desire to drink appeared in a vacuum. That was how it felt, because I didn't understand the think → feel → act cycle. But my desire to drink hadn't always been with me (and neither has yours). I wasn't born wanting a drink to quell social anxiety. I learned the behavior in college.

The key then, is to roll back the tape and figure out the thought that is generating the desire to drink. It seems almost too obvious to be useful. But your other option is to play whack-a-mole with the desire to drink. Every time it surfaces you can bash it over the head with willpower in an effort to resist drinking. Doesn't that sound exhausting? Or you can begin the work of identifying the thought that triggers the desire and work at changing it. The think → feel → act cycle gave me an entirely new framework for change.

Understanding that the think → feel → act cycle is always working in the background of your brain and that your actions aren't driven by a mysterious, unknowable force, is key to bringing an unconscious habit into consciousness. This work takes time, but it's the best way to unravel your desire to drink.

You're Thinking Thoughts All Day Long

Every day, you think tens of thousands of thoughts about yourself, your world, and the situations and people you encounter. Anyone that has tried to meditate knows just how numerous our thoughts are. They're like an electronic news ticker constantly running through your mind. You can experience this right now. Set a timer for one minute and try to focus only on your breathing. Don't think about anything else, just try to stay present and notice the rise and fall of your chest. Go ahead; try it.

Did your mind wander? Did you find yourself thinking about something other than your breathing? Most people do. Your brain is always thinking. In fact, most of us have gotten so used to the steady stream of thoughts that run through our minds that this chatter just becomes the background noise of our lives. It's like having the TV on while sitting in front of your computer. After a while, you might forget that the TV is even there.

If you're going to harness the think → feel → act cycle, you need to pay close attention to what you're thinking. The problem is, when most of my clients tune into their thoughts they don't like what they hear. It's the think → feel → act cycle in action: think a negative thought and you'll feel a negative emotion. Most people get stuck here because they are missing a crucial piece of information: **you are not your thoughts**. How do you know this? Because you can observe the electronic news ticker in your mind, and if part of you can *observe* your thoughts, then part of you is also *separate* from your thoughts. This is why it's possible to observe what we're thinking, notice its effect on us, and, most importantly, learn how to change it.

When we believe that our thoughts are "who we are" we feel helpless when confronted with our negative thinking. Consider this. What would happen if someone followed you around criticizing everything you do? At first, it would probably be annoying. Maybe you'd roll your eyes and tell yourself to ignore the criticisms. If they kept at it, you might get so frustrated that you'd yell at them to stop. But what if they didn't? Soon you'd devise plans to escape. If that didn't work, you might eventually try to find things that would help muffle the sound of their voice so that their opinions, while still there, didn't sound quite so loud.

These are all things we do with our own negative thinking. We tell ourselves to ignore it. We yell at ourselves to stop. We try to run away from our thoughts. Finally, if we get in the habit of using alcohol as a crutch, we use a drink to numb ourselves. We feel bombarded by our thinking because we believe it is outside of our control. No one ever showed us the think → feel → act cycle in action or how to use the cycle to our advantage. Instead, we assume that the way we think is fixed. Our thoughts are just "who we are," they aren't optional. We miss the opportunity to make the connection between the way we think, the way we feel, and the way we act, as well as how much power we have to harness this cycle.

Your Thoughts are Always Optional

Intellectually, the think → feel → act cycle makes sense to most people. Where it gets sticky is when you start applying it to your own life. When I was first introduced to the concept and the idea that all I needed to do was change my thoughts if I wanted to feel better and stop over-drinking, I was not amused. In fact, I felt like screaming, "So I'm just supposed to snap my fingers and start thinking differently and then I'll magically solve this problem? Don't you think if it were that easy I would have done that by now?"

I knew that I had a boatload of negative thoughts. I knew that these thoughts sucked. I knew that I shouldn't be so critical of myself or beat myself up. The problem was I didn't have the first clue how to feel good about myself, and the suggestion that I should just "change my thoughts" infuriated me. The think → feel → act cycle felt like one big game of pin-the-blame-on-Rachel. It was especially frustrating when I realized I was using alcohol to cover up the negative feelings that my own thoughts had created.

The very fact that so many people hate spending time alone without anything to distract themselves is an indication to some degree that most people intuitively understand that their thoughts create feelings. When left to your own devices, you may avoid sitting by yourself because so much of what runs through your mind is terrible. You don't like being alone with your thoughts because so many of them are negative. You may feel like crap when left to your own devices. Hence, you try to distract yourself so you won't have to be alone with your thoughts.

Most people aren't used to examining their thoughts from a distance or considering that with practice they can be optional. Rather, we assume what we think is true. For example, if I think I'm a failure, then I must actually be one. If I think I'm ugly, then it's also true. Maybe you've even defended these thoughts to another person ("No really, I'm a failure. Let me prove it to you….").

It's not surprising then that learning about the think → feel → act cycle can provoke resistance at first. Here are some of the most common reactions I get from clients.

- **"Yeah, yeah I've heard this all before. Say nice stuff about yourself. I've tried using affirmations, and it doesn't work."** Simply, the think → feel → act cycle isn't about affirmations it's about understanding why you feel and act the way you do. Blindly reciting positive statements about yourself usually doesn't work. Do you know why? What if I told you to repeat to yourself, "The world is flat" 10 times a day. Do you think you'd believe the world is flat by the end of the month? I doubt it. Because you truly believe that the world is round. Reciting "The world is flat" over and over isn't going to convince you otherwise. Changing your thoughts requires practicing *believable* replacement, and most affirmations you read about are so positive they feel totally out of reach.

- **"If my thoughts create my feelings then it's my fault when I feel bad?"** For starters, just because you understand the think → feel → act cycle doesn't mean you can put it into action right away. This is a totally new concept that will take practice to master. I wish I had learned this when I was in grade school, but I didn't, and I doubt you did either. Shifting your worldview about what creates your feelings is no small task, especially since we're surrounded by messages that our happiness is found in our external environment. It's not enough to intellectually understand the think → feel → act cycle; you have to see it in action in your own life before you can start to harness it.

• **"What about if I do something really embarrassing when I'm drunk? You're telling me I should just pretend not to care?"** I'm not suggesting you turn a blind eye to behavior that isn't serving you, but how many times have you replayed a scene you regretted over and over in you mind all the while saying to yourself, "I'm such an idiot." Maybe you really do believe that whatever you did is idiotic, but how is the thought, "I'm such an idiot" serving you? The more you keep thinking this thought, the more your shame grows. The more shame you feel, the more likely you are to return to a trusted coping mechanism that can help you forget how you feel—having a drink. Framing your behavior as stupid or idiotic may feel true, but it only ever creates feelings that keep you stuck. Getting to a better place isn't about pretending nothing is wrong; it's about finding a way to extend compassion and kindness when you are at your lowest.

• **"Sticking with my decision not to drink wouldn't be so difficult if my friend/boyfriend/husband wasn't making me feel bad about it."** Understanding that other people don't create your feelings is so important when it comes to drinking because too often we tell ourselves that it's just easier to have a drink and blend in rather than face questions and judgment from others. Most of us spend a lot of time and energy trying to get everyone in our lives to act differently so we can feel better. The trouble is that while you may have some influence over other people, ultimately you're not the one in control of how they act. You are free to pin your happiness on someone else's behavior, but if you do you will be at their mercy. The think → feel → act cycle turns out to be really useful in these situations. Instead of spending your energy on changing their behavior (something which you cannot control), you can focus your attention where you do have control: pinpointing the thoughts that are creating your feelings and working to change them. One of my all-time favorite questions to uncover your thinking about another person's behavior is, "What am I making this mean?"

- **"How I think is just my personality, and I'm not going to be a Pollyanna."** Shifting your mindset does not mean changing who you are or assuming a different personality. Nor is the goal of this work to be happy 100 percent of the time or only see the bright side of everything. Shifting your mindset is about becoming comfortable feeling the full range of human emotions (a crucial step if you want to stop using alcohol as a crutch). This work will help you feel happier more often, but you must also be able to sit with emotions like jealously, grief, frustration, anger, sadness, and shame rather than needing something to dull every negative emotion. The good news is that the think → feel → act cycle shows you how to handle and change them without turning to alcohol.

The most important thing to remember is that part of changing how you think is practicing noticing that your thoughts are optional. This is not something you've practiced so far. What you've spent years practicing is the unconscious thoughts, "If I think something, it's true"; "This is the way I am"; "I can't change the way I feel"; or "This is just how I think about this person/situation/event." You have unknowingly practiced the belief that your thoughts and your feelings are not within your control.

The think → feel → act cycle flies in the face of what our culture conditions us to believe: that our external environment creates how we feel. It's why we spend so much time and energy wishing that our jobs were better, our bodies were thinner, our families were more understanding, our romantic partners were more supportive, and our bank accounts were bigger. We have been taught that these are the things that keep us from being happy. It's the same reason why so many people preoccupy themselves with finding the perfect job, losing weight, trying to get their family or their partner to act a certain way, or fantasizing about winning the lottery. We've all been told that these are the things that will finally make us happy. The think → feel → act cycle points us in a different direction. Happiness is not the result of everything you have in life, but your mindset.

Separating Facts from Opinions

How do you start this process? **You have to learn to notice what you're thinking and begin the process of distinguishing between the events in your life and your opinion of them.** This is harder than it sounds, but being able to do so shows you where you can intervene in the think → feel → act cycle. To begin with, most of us aren't used to observing our thoughts—in fact, you might have more practice tuning them out. But once you start noticing what you're thinking, you can start understanding why you feel the way you do and, if you want, how to begin the process of changing this feeling. This is key if you want to use the think → feel → act cycle to reduce your desire to drink or stop using alcohol to numb how you feel.

Back to Epictetus, the philosopher living in ancient Greece who said, "Men are disturbed *not* by the things that happen, but by their *opinion* of the things that happen." Think back to the weather example in Chapter 2. The rainy day itself doesn't dictate how you feel; your thoughts about the rain do. You've been conditioned to believe the opposite—that everything around you creates your feelings—and that the cycle looks like this: life happens → feel → act. Notice what's missing? Your thoughts. It will take time to switch to a new perspective on the world (life happens → *think* → feel → act) and untangle what is happening in your life (the facts) from your opinions (your thoughts).

The things that happen in your life are the facts. They are the objective realities of your world stripped of any judgment or opinion. This includes things like other people, the weather, the political climate, the past, your weight, your appearance, your job, your bank account, your relationship, etc. Every fact is neutral until you have a thought about it. Intuitively, you may already have an inkling that this is the case because you've seen how no two people react exactly the same way to the same set of circumstances or life events. Most people chalk it up to personality instead of understanding the role of their thoughts.

You have to practice separating out the facts from your opinion of the facts if you want to begin watching how the think → feel → act cycle plays out in your life. Until you can see the cycle in action, it will be difficult to harness it for change. Let's take a look at a couple of examples.

Let's say that two people come into $5,000 inheritances—that's the fact. The size of the check is neutral. Neither person has an emotional response to the money until thinking about it. Their opinions may be wildly divergent depending on their judgments about the fact. For example, one person might think she hit the jackpot and feel excited; whereas, someone else might think this check is peanuts and feel disappointed. What matters (and what creates unique emotional responses) is not the inheritance itself but what each person thinks about it.

Perhaps you think that their emotional reactions (excitement versus disappointment) are dependent on how much money each person currently has in the bank, and by extension are not really in their control. For example, someone who makes minimum wage will probably think that $5,000 is a lot of money, but a millionaire will shrug her shoulders at the size of the check. What if the person who makes minimum wage was expecting five times that amount from his grandmother's will? He might look at the check for $5,000 and feel angry because he believes he was cheated. What if the millionaire made her fortune by being excessively frugal? She might be excited because she thinks that every penny counts. The point is, neither the $5,000 nor your bank statements create your feelings. Your emotional response depends on what you think.

What does this have to do with your drinking? When you use alcohol as a crutch, it's because you unconsciously teach your brain that it makes a specific situation easier or a part of your life more bearable. Essentially, you're using alcohol to give yourself relief from a negative emotion. Because negative emotions are always caused by your thoughts, in order to find a better means of coping you need to pay attention to your thinking. If you want to change how you feel you have to be aware of your thoughts and aware that they are creating how you feel. To do this you must be able to distinguish fact from opinion.

Here's another example: body shame. Body shame is important to consider because so many women have the experience of walking into a party and immediately scanning the room to see how they measure up. If they feel self-conscious, they might get into the habit of using a couple of drinks to take the edge off how they are feeling. For many women, the thoughts we have in social settings intensify our negative feelings about the way we look, and having a drink is welcome relief.

I know this firsthand. My self-consciousness and anxiety always started when I was getting ready to go out. Everything I saw in the mirror was wrong. I couldn't find anything I looked good in. My skin was a mess. I hated my hair. Before I even walked out the door, I was a wreck. By the time I got to the party, my brain was primed to scan the room and see how I measured up. My assessment was always the same: I couldn't compare. Here I was, trying to have fun, and I felt intensely insecure and self-conscious. In college, I learned a quick and easy solution. With enough of a buzz, I started to forget about feeling insecure and awkward. Once I was drinking, I stopped comparing myself to every other woman in the room.

I didn't realize two crucial things. First, what was creating my anxiety and insecurity was not the way I looked or what I saw in the mirror. The way I felt was created by what I thought about my appearance. Second, everything I was thinking was optional. I believed that all my thoughts about my appearance—"Everything in the mirror is wrong." "I don't look good in anything." "My skin is a mess." "I hate my hair."—were just facts and not the least bit optional. After all, they certainly felt true. But the facts were only this: I had a body, skin, hair, and clothing. The rest of it was judgment. I didn't yet understand the power of the think → feel → act cycle and believed the only way to change how I felt was to either work harder at being attractive or get drunk and forget about how I felt. I didn't yet understand the role of my thoughts.

I don't know a single woman who hasn't at some point in her life struggled with body shame. Most of us think what I did: the solution to feeling good about how we look is just to lose weight, fix our skin, tame our hair. We jump on the hamster wheel of never-ending self-improvement, hoping that changing what we see in the mirror will be the thing that finally makes us feel better.

Most women also have the opposite experience. We reach our "goal weight" and move our attention to another part of our bodies that needs to be "fixed." In my twenties, I was at my lowest weight, I finally cleared up my skin, and mastered my curly hair. Did I feel beautiful? Nope. Was I finally free of hating my body and how I looked? Not at all. I turned around and found new "problem areas" to fixate on. I remember this every time that body shame starts to creep back in and tries to convince me I need to lose weight. Back when I was at my then "goal weight," I didn't feel confident about how I looked. It was the chorus of negative thoughts—not the number on the scale or the image in the mirror—determined how I felt. The same is true today. If I want to feel confident in my appearance, I need to be aware of my thoughts and practice my thinking. Back then, the only way I knew how to feel confident and sexy and forget about my hang-ups was to down a couple of drinks. I didn't understand that the shame I experienced around my appearance wasn't the result of my weight, or my hair, or my skin, or my outfit, but my *thoughts* about all of these things.

Most women can relate to having a friend who, in their mind, has the body they dream of. "If only I had her body, I could stop worrying about how I look all the time and feel good about myself." But you've probably listened to that same friend complain about her appearance. You think she's being crazy. You'd kill to have her stomach, her legs, her breasts and yet here she is unsatisfied with them, and no amount of convincing from you changes her mind. In fact, how many times has someone complimented the way you look only for you to immediately dismiss his or her opinion? This is yet another example of the think → feel → act cycle and the fact that your feelings are created by your thoughts. If your external environment created your emotions, then the compliments you get from other people would always make you feel happy.

I was on this merry-go-round with one of my good friends in college. To me, she had the perfect body. If I looked like her, I wouldn't need the help of liquid confidence when I walked into a party (at least that's what I told myself). She, on the other hand, would complain about her thighs. This was crazy to me. Yet I could not convince her that she had the perfect body, and she could not convince me that she needed to lose weight. The only fact here was that my friend had a body. But the only thing that mattered (and determined how she felt) was her opinion of it. Her thoughts caused her to look at her body with derision while my thoughts made me look at it with jealousy.

This is why understanding the think → feel → act cycle is so important and why noticing your thoughts is the first step. How you feel—including when you look in the mirror—is always the result of how you think, and it works like this with *everything*, from the mundane to the extraordinary. When I finally understood this concept, it was revelatory. But it was also a difficult pill to swallow, especially when it came to my drinking. I knew I was using alcohol as a crutch to feel less awkward, insecure, and self-conscious, but it was frustrating to realize that my thoughts were unknowingly creating the very emotions I was trying to run from.

No one had ever taught me that my thoughts created my feelings, that my thoughts were optional, and that I could practice thinking thoughts on purpose. I was blind to how the cycle worked. Here's the good news.

- **Your thoughts are the one thing that no one can ever force you to change. You're in charge, and with practice you can change them if you want.**
- **Even small tweaks in how you think can have an outsized impact on how you feel.** (More on this in Chapter 8.)

Your work is to start noticing your thoughts and learning to separate out the facts from your opinions. As soon as you can distinguish between the two, you'll begin to understand what's causing you to feel the way you do. You'll also be able to see that your thoughts are optional and that you can choose to practice thinking something different. Once you have this basic awareness and are good at untangling facts from your opinions, you can begin the process of changing how you feel.

A great way to practice this skill is by getting your thoughts out of your head and onto a piece of paper (I'll show you how in the following exercise). Putting your thoughts on paper helps you practice observing your thoughts with some distance. The first time someone suggested that I make a daily practice of writing down my thoughts, I was not having it. I already knew my thinking was terrible. I was bombarded by negative thoughts about myself all day long. Why would I want to reinforce my thinking by putting it on paper? I thought that turning the volume up on my thoughts, especially when so many of them were so negative, would only make me feel worse. If anything, I wanted someone to tell me how to get them to shut up, rather than open the floodgates.

Gaining awareness of what you're thinking, and how it fits into the think → feel → act cycle is the first step. Especially when you're used to using alcohol to tune out your thoughts, you need to make a habit of tuning in. Making a daily practice of getting your thoughts out of your head and onto paper, and then looking at them objectively is the best practice you can do. It's not only a crucial step in transforming your mindset, but down the road it will help you start changing how you feel. After all, you can't break a thought pattern unless you're fully conscious of it.

Exercise 2: Observing Your Thoughts

Time Required: 10 minutes

There are two parts to this exercise: First, you'll record your thoughts onto a piece of paper, and then you'll examine what you wrote and distinguish between the facts and your opinions.

This exercise sounds deceptively simple, but it can be quite challenging at first, especially when you come across thoughts that you've unknowingly practiced thinking over and over again. For example, you might think "I'm a screw-up" is a fact because it feels utterly true to you. You might be able to cite reams of evidence in support of the mistakes you've made. Maybe you've convinced yourself that the only way to not think this thought is to step into a time machine and change the past.

"I'm a screw up" is not a fact. It is not neutral, nor is it free of judgment. Think about how the thought "I'm a screw-up" works in the think → feel → act cycle. What emotion do you think it produces? Shame? Embarrassment? Resignation? When you feel one of these emotions, how do you think you're likely to act? Do you put yourself out there and try new things? Do you stick with something even when it gets hard? Or do you tell yourself there's no point in even trying?

Making a regular practice of emptying the thoughts in your head onto a piece of paper will help you start to watch the think → feel → act cycle unfold instead of being caught up in it. It will also help you practice being curious with yourself and what you're thinking.

This exercise is not the same as writing in a journal. When you write in a journal your tendency is to *describe* what's happening in your life. You probably also edit yourself. You think about what to write and put together a coherent story. So much so, that someone who doesn't know you could probably pick up your diary and at least follow along.

In this exercise, you are trying to capture your stream of consciousness. Your thoughts may not be connected to each other. Side by side on a piece of paper, they may not make a lot of sense. That's okay. Your goal is to observe the thoughts on your "electronic news ticker" not write a coherent story. The more you observe, the more you can start to change the think → feel → act cycle in ways that help you.

You can use this exercise in two different ways:

- **Record what you're thinking first thing in the morning**: use this time as an opportunity to see what's going on in your mind before the day's events unfold. Morning is ideal for this exercise, but any time of day will work.
- **Record what you're thinking when you have the urge to drink**: I'll discuss this more in Chapter 5, but this is a great exercise to help you start to understand the thinking that is

triggering your urge to drink. If you use this exercise *before* acting on the urge, it can also help you practice not acting immediately on every urge.

Follow these steps:

- **Set a timer for two minutes. On a piece of paper write down everything that you're thinking**. Remember you aren't journaling. You're trying to capture your stream of consciousness. What you write might seem disjointed or unconnected. Don't edit yourself. Include any thoughts that seem silly or irrelevant.
- **Keep your pen moving.** Don't think about what you "should" write; just write. If nothing comes up, just keep writing, "I don't know what I'm thinking" over and over again. Your thoughts will eventually surface if you keep your pen moving.
- **As you write down your thoughts, try to be curious rather than judgmental.** The temptation is always to start judging what you're thinking. You might find yourself not wanting to write a thought down because it's "stupid" or you know you "shouldn't" think this way. Once you start judging your thoughts you'll start editing yourself, and you'll miss the full picture of what you're thinking. Pay particular attention to any thoughts you resist putting on paper.

At the end of two minutes, spend the remaining eight minutes examining what you wrote and trying to separate the facts from your opinion.

- **Circle the facts:** If you're having trouble identifying what a fact looks like, scan for nouns (body, boss, boyfriend, job, house, checkout line, etc.) or events or actions (ate, spoke, sex, work, clean, stand). Anything that appears neutral.

- **Underline your thoughts**: If you're having trouble identifying what is an opinion, look for any judgments. Often you can spot them in the adjectives and adverbs you use to describe the nouns (fat, jerk, selfish, horrible, messy, slow, etc.).

The goal is to start practicing separating the facts from your opinions. This will help you learn what is optional and where you can intervene in the think → feel → act cycle. It takes practice. You might find yourself trying to justify your opinions. That's always a good sign. When you find yourself saying, "Well sure that's my opinion, but *everyone* would agree with me" or "If you know so-so you'd think this too," it means you've hit on a thought that's particularly sticky for you. Even if you believe 99.9 percent of the world would be on board with your assessment of events, it's still an opinion, which means it's always optional.

Below is a sample thought download from a client so you can begin to see what is an objective fact and what is a subjective interpretation.

I can't believe I got so drunk last night. I told myself I would have two beers and ended up having six. What was I thinking? I'm so ashamed of myself. Why did I get so drunk? What is wrong me? Why am I always such a screw-up? I can't believe I said that to Sam. I'm so humiliated. This exercise is stupid. I have real things I need to do. I don't know what to write. I don't know what to write. I don't know what to write. I hate this. I don't want this to be my life. I just wish that I was like everyone else.

Are you able to separate the facts from the thoughts? Remember what Epictetus said: "Men are disturbed *not* by the things that happen, but by their opinion of the things that happen."

- The thing that happened: I drank six beers and said something to Sam.
- My opinion of what happened: Everything else in the paragraph.

The point of doing this is not to say that I *shouldn't* have been ashamed or humiliated or embarrassed. Nor is it to turn a blind eye to the things that aren't working in your life and act as if everything is fabulous. The point of this is to understand how your thinking—and not what happened—is causing you to feel ashamed, humiliated, and embarrassed.

It seems difficult because you're probably reasoning, "Well, I just got drunk and embarrassed myself so how else should I feel?" But the point is to understand that your emotions are not caused by what happened—having six beers and saying something to Sam. They're caused by what you think of what happened. You know this because you can see that it is hypothetically possible to have different thoughts about what happened. For example, "I wish I hadn't said that to Sam but it's not the end of the world" or "I made a mistake, but I can see my way through this." Those thoughts may not be available to you right now, but they might be with practice, and they will certainly feel better.

Think about it this way. When you feel ashamed, humiliated, and embarrassed, how do you act? You probably isolate yourself and keep thinking the same thoughts over and over until you're overwhelmed. After a while, going out and having a drink might not seem like such a bad idea—at least it would help you forget what happened and give you some relief. If on the other hand, you understand that your thoughts create how you feel, you would at least have the framework for how to move yourself to a better place without wishing you could build a time machine and change the past. After a night when you drank more than you intended, you're only going to compound the problem by relentlessly beating yourself up. You want to figure out a way to pick yourself up and figure out how to change what isn't serving you rather than staying stuck in emotions that make the situation worse and might end up causing you to drink more. It takes practice, but it's possible when you understand the think → feel → act cycle.

Being able to notice your thoughts and get some distance from them takes time. Don't expect that you'll be able to do this overnight. It takes practice. The more skilled you become at this practice, the better able you will be to identify your opinions as they appear and change the think → feel → act cycle before it takes hold. Not only that, but soon you'll be able to actually create the way you want to feel just by practicing thinking new thoughts (More on that in Chapter 8).

The Invisible Stories Around You

Now that you understand the difference between the facts and your opinion of the facts and have clarity on the two, you may start to wonder, "Why the heck do I think this way?" especially when you notice that:

- Some of your thoughts are decidedly unhelpful, especially the ones that trigger the very behavior you are trying to change, and
- There are certain negative thoughts that you seem to think *all* the time.

It's important to remember that your thoughts about yourself and the environment around you did not appear in a vacuum. From the moment you were born, your brain was surrounded by stories. Stories are the vehicle by which humans try to make sense of what they see and experience, pass on information, teach lessons, and generally attempt to apply some order to the chaos that is the world. Stories tell us about our past, our present, and our future, and are created for purely entertainment value or for a distinct moral purpose. All stories have one thing in common: they are based on someone's subjective interpretation, or simply their thoughts.

Why do you need to understand this? Knowing that some of your most unhelpful thoughts didn't just appear but are influenced by the stories around you can bring a little bit of relief. Once you can see that the lens through which you see yourself, understand your problems, and view the world is influenced by the previously invisible stories around you, you can start understanding why you think the way you do rather than beating yourself up for thinking unhelpful thoughts.

Here's the fascinating part: you are *unconsciously absorbing* stories from your environment all the time. They come from the media, your family, your friends, books, movies, magazines, music, you name it. You're surrounded by stories—in particular, stories concerning alcohol and people who struggle with it. These stories influence your own think → feel → act cycle in positive and negative ways Here are some common stories you may have unknowingly picked up about drinking:

- **Everyone wants to drink, it's just that some people can't.** This goes right along with the thought, "If I could drink, I would drink, but I can't." It assumes that desire for alcohol is a constant that is unchangeable. You'll always have it. Your desire will never leave you. You can decide to stop drinking, but you can't decide to stop desiring it. (As you've seen from the think → feel → act cycle, our thoughts, not the world around us, create our emotions, including desire.)
- **You can't change unless you hit rock bottom.** This story is widely accepted, but when you think about it, it doesn't make much logical sense. How on earth can anyone know where their "bottom" is? The only way to do so would be to look into the future to confirm that they will never be as low as they are in

the moment. The problem with this story is that it implies that change is only possible in the depths of despair. When I was struggling I remember thinking, "Maybe things just haven't gotten bad enough for me to be ready to change." Wouldn't it be more helpful to think that change is possible at any moment?

- **People who drink too much lack willpower.** Let's be honest. Have you ever eaten a bowl of ice cream when you were on a diet? Have you purchased something you couldn't really afford? Have you ever promised yourself that you could skip working out today if you go for a run tomorrow, only to have a week go by before you lace up your shoes again? All people make decisions that they don't stick to. It's not unique to people who overdrink. When we focus on willpower alone, we miss the important role of the think → feel → act cycle.

These are just three of the invisible stories around you that affect how you think about alcohol. Looking at your thoughts is just one piece of the puzzle. These stories contribute to how you feel about your struggle, whether you believe you can succeed at change, and many times whether you seek support. As such, you also need to identify the stories you have about alcohol, both positive and negative, and see them for what they are: helpful or unhelpful thoughts.

Alcohol has been around for thousands of years, so it is no surprise that all of us are surrounded by stories about what drinking and not drinking means. These will vary depending on the specific environment in which you grew up and your life experiences, but here were some of the common ones I had:

- Drinking is normal. Everybody does it.
- Drinking makes everything more fun.
- People who don't drink are boring and uptight.

- Everybody hates a buzz-kill.
- Some people can't trust themselves around alcohol.
- Once you're sober, a single drop can set you back.

Now you may read this list and think, "This doesn't sound right for me." There's never a single list that applies to everyone. The point is to take the time to consider what your stories about alcohol are. Your decision about your struggle and whether you want to keep drinking, moderate, or stop altogether is influenced by your stories about what drinking means. You can list the pros and cons of your drinking; but if you fail to identify the stories you have, it's difficult to fully understand what's really driving your decisions. It's also why so many people say they feel ambivalent about the decision to stop drinking. They are fully aware of the negative repercussions, but they have a lot of unconscious negative stories about what stopping will mean about who they are and their life going forward.

What usually happens is that you have stories running in the background and you don't even realize that they are optional stories. Like all your other thoughts, you just see them as facts. "If I quit drinking, I'll stop being fun." "If I stop drinking, dating will be impossible." "If I stop drinking, I'll always be the odd-man out." The list goes on. You see these thoughts as facts rather than opinion in part because you've thought them repeatedly and in part because you've unknowingly created a lot of evidence to back them up. You've probably spent easily a decade connecting going out to dinner, hanging out with friends, and having fun with drinking. Of course, you'll have a hard time believing that life could be fun if you take a break from drinking.

Ultimately, you must be able to identify your stories about drinking and understand how they contribute to your own think $\rightarrow$ feel $\rightarrow$ act cycle. You must be able to see what is an optional opinion, even in the face of lots of evidence. Your stories contribute to what you're making your struggle mean (e.g., "something is wrong with you") and what you think life will be like without alcohol (e.g., "life will suck"). Identifying your stories will help you understand why you feel ambivalent about change.

Exercise 3: Identify Your Stories about Alcohol

Time Required: 30 minutes—1 hour

Identifying your stories about drinking can help you understand why you feel ambivalent about taking a break from drinking. Listing the pros and cons is a good start, but it's difficult to fully understand what is driving your decision if you don't at the same time also understand the unconscious stories that influence you.

Complete these sentences and to uncover your beliefs around drinking.

- **People who drink are....**
- **People who don't like to drink are....**
- **People who choose not to drink are....**
- **People who can't control how much they drink are....**
- **Drinking is necessary for....**
- **Drinking makes things....**
- **Drinking makes me....**
- **Drinking makes other people....**
- **Drinking makes meeting people....**
- **Drinking makes dating....**
- **Life without alcohol would be....**
- **If I can't drink normally, it means....**
- **My greatest worry or fear about stopping drinking is....**
- **I would be happier if I could....**

I want you to go back and read through these statements. Do any of them seem optional? Arc you willing to challenge any of these assumptions? You'll want to return to this exercise as you make your way through the other tools in the book.

4   The Role of Your Emotions

Why Do You Drink?

People drink for lots of different reasons. To take away stress and anxiety, forget about being lonely, to relieve themselves of boredom, or dull their pain. They might like that a drink makes them energized or that it helps them fall asleep. People use alcohol to open up, meet people, fit in, and broach difficult conversations. They use alcohol to soothe their tears and to celebrate their joy.

It all boils down to this: people drink because they want to feel a certain way. It makes a lot of sense then that alcohol is often used as a crutch to dull discomfort because drinking can temporarily change how we feel. Remember, something becomes a crutch when you unconsciously teach your brain that it makes a specific situation easier or a part of your life more bearable, usually because you don't have alternative means to cope with discomfort. For most people, negative emotions are their primary source of discomfort.

If you don't believe me, just think about how much time and energy you've spent trying to get happy, the lengths that you've gone to acquire this feeling. It's not just because happy feels so good; it's because most people have a terrible relationship with their negative emotions. Most people don't ever want negative emotions in their life; they just want to make them to go away.

Alcohol is a quick and easy fix when you're looking to feel differently, especially when you want to get rid of a negative emotion. Once you have enough of a buzz, whatever you were feeling before you picked up a glass lessens. Alcohol has numbed, dulled, and quieted the feeling. When you don't understand what creates your emotions, or how to change them, it's no wonder having a drink can become people's go-to solution when they want to feel better.

Learning how to stop using alcohol as a crutch depends on learning how to have a different relationship with your emotions. If you can learn how not to run from these feelings, then you won't need alcohol to dull them. The trick is to change how you view emotions. Every emotion you have is just your body's way of trying to tell you something. They're a non-verbal alert system that can tune you into what you need, if only you'll pause and listen.

A lot of my clients find the idea of needing to familiarize themselves with their emotions ludicrous. They're already plenty familiar with feeling lonely, anxious, insecure, and depressed, thank you very much. Negative emotions are a part of their everyday life. They feel them all the damn time.

If you want to skip this chapter because you "know all about your feelings," I get it. But stay with me. The power in this work is learning how to distinguish between each step of the think → feel → act process. The finer you parse between the two, the more able you will be to control and change the cycle. Feeling in control and able to handle whatever comes your way requires that you aren't at the mercy of a cycle that you don't fully understand.

What Are Emotions Anyway?

Emotions aren't a paragraph of thoughts or even a single sentence. Emotions are a one-word feeling state: happy, angry, sad, jealous, bored, lonely, excited, nervous, anxious, guilty, regretful. While I'm sure you've felt all of these emotions at one time in your life, the real question is how do you know you're experiencing an emotion? The answer is you feel it in your body.

All emotions manifest physically in your body. You may not be practiced at describing the physical sensations that accompany emotions, but you're already familiar with the concept. You have butterflies in your stomach when you're nervous. Your heart swells when you feel pride. Fear causes a shiver to run down your spine, or you go weak in the knees with desire. Depending on the emotion you're experiencing, your breathing slows down or speeds up, your muscles tense or relax, and different parts of your body flush, feel cold, or have other sensations.

Most people pay very little attention to the physical manifestations of an emotion. If they do notice, it's usually only when an emotion comes on very strong. But every emotion, no matter its intensity, has its own accompanying physical manifestations. You've just gotten so used to tangling up your emotions and your thoughts that you think about an emotion as something that happens only in your mind and often miss what is happening in your body.

To become familiar with your emotions, you need to begin the practice of learning how to describe how they feel in your body. Remember, if you're using alcohol as a crutch, it's because you're trying to escape discomfort, and the discomfort we are most often trying to avoid is the discomfort associated with a negative emotion. Once you start paying attention to the physical manifestations happening in your body, the question becomes, what makes tingling, sweating, flushing, etc. so intolerable that you'll do anything to avoid it?

Too touchy-feely for you? Hang in there with me, because there is a huge benefit to learning how to describe the way emotions feel in your body. The more able you are to stay present with your emotions, rather than escaping them, the less you'll need alcohol to take the edge off or numb how you're feeling.

Separating Emotions from Thoughts

The first step is making sure you're really clear about separating your thoughts from your emotions. Usually when I ask clients what they are feeling, I get one of two answers. Sometimes it tumbles out in one big story. Here's an example from my client, Claudia:

> *I feel so stupid. I spent the last year and a half putting my life on hold and trying to be the best girlfriend I could be to prove that he should care about me. I ignored all the signs telling me that this guy was not ready or interested in a relationship. As soon as I started drinking, I knew I couldn't keep it in anymore. I had to tell him how I really felt. Of course, he reacted terribly and we got in a huge drunken fight. He said he doesn't think we work together. If I hadn't gotten drunk and had just kept my mouth shut, none of this would have happened. I'm such an idiot.*

Other times, the response I get to "What are you feeling?" is shorter:

I feel terrible.
I feel like crap.
I feel all the feelings.
I don't know.

Did you see any emotions in any of the examples? I'm sure when you read Claudia's story you could feel what this woman was going through. She was clearly upset because her boyfriend had dumped her. That much is clear, but did she list a single emotion? Nope. Most people do the same thing. Instead of pinpointing the specific emotion they're feeling, they list a bunch of thoughts.

Happy. Angry. Sad. Jealous. Bored. Lonely. Excited. Nervous. Anxious. Guilty. Regretful. These are emotions. If you can't identify the specific emotional state, it's actually harder for you to unwind the think → feel → act cycle. Remember, this is the cycle that drives everything, so you want to get good at parsing out each step so that you can ultimately work to change it.

It can be frustrating for someone when I push her to get specific on the exact emotion that she is feeling. She knows she feels terrible. Isn't that enough? It all goes back to the think → feel → act cycle. Remember, most people operate from a place that looks like this: life happens → feel → act. They assume that everything happening in their external environment creates how they feel. Not only do they miss the role of their thoughts, but they confuse their thoughts with their emotions.

Here's what I mean. Go back to that first example, when Claudia was suffering after a break up. For the sake of argument, let's say she feels sad (There's clearly a host of other potential emotions going on here, but for now, let's stick with sad). If you were to ask her, "Why do you feel sad" what do you think her answer would be? Probably something along the lines of, "Because I got drunk, told my boyfriend how I felt, and he dumped me." This is obvious, right? A series of events unfolded, and because of them she's sad.

Because we don't understand the role of our thoughts and have our thoughts and our emotions tangled together, we spend a lot of energy trying to change our external world in order to feel better. Here's what most people would suggest to Claudia so that she could feel better:

- Go out and party and forget how you feel.
- Apologize to your ex and maybe he'll take you back.
- Meet someone else—that will take your mind off your ex.
- Commiserate with a friend about what a jerk he is.
- Curl up on the couch with a pint of ice cream and binge-watch Netflix.
- Take a trip and try to take your mind off everything.
- Keep yourself busy so you don't dwell on how you feel.
- Hope that time will do its thing, and after a while you won't feel this way anymore.

These are standard suggestions, but they all focus on the idea that Claudia's external world is going to make her feel better. By getting her ex back, finding a new one, getting a friend to agree he's a jerk, distracting herself from how she feels, or letting time run its course.

The framework for this thinking is simple: something in her life happened which made her feel a certain way, so to feel better she needs to change what is happening in her life. What I'm offering is something different. It's the idea that you can use the think → feel → act cycle to understand why you feel the way you do and ultimately change it. It's not the fact that her boyfriend dumped her that created her emotions; it's what she is thinking about these events (or back to my favorite question from Chapter 3, "What are you making it mean?"). The way Claudia feels is a result of what she *thinks* about the fact that she was dumped, and not the fact that her boyfriend dumped her. Did I really just say that? Yes, I did. Maybe you're thinking something along these lines right now:

So you're blaming Claudia for feeling sad? That's crazy! She was just dumped. Maybe the guy is a real jerk. Maybe she really loved him. Maybe he treated her like crap? Maybe she shouldn't have gotten drunk and started a fight. But the idea that you should just slap a smile on your face and pretend it doesn't hurt when someone breaks your heart is ludicrous.

Let me be really clear. Just because her thoughts create her feelings doesn't mean that Claudia shouldn't feel sad or that she should even feel different. This work is not about feeling happy all the time. The think → feel → act cycle is about understanding that if your thoughts are the reason why you feel the way you do in every moment, then it is also the way out of whatever you are feeling. You don't have to wait for things in your external environment to change. You can start laying the groundwork to feel better now. You're in control.

Here's the paradox: Just because your thoughts create your feelings does not mean that you should always be content. For starters, I don't want to live like that. I want to feel the full range of human emotions. I want to grieve when I lose someone I love. I want to be angry when I see injustices in the world. I want to feel longing for the people I miss. I want to feel discomfort when I'm testing my boundaries. I want to feel the full spectrum of emotions because they carry essential information. My emotions are indications of what I'm thinking and by extension useful windows into what is happening in my mind.

Not only that, but when I'm stuck in a moment where the only thing that comes out of my mouth is—*I feel terrible. I feel like crap. I feel all the feelings. I don't know.*—I want a pathway forward. I want to be able to identify the emotion I am feeling so that I can pinpoint the thought that is creating it. This at least gives me some direction for how to feel better. No matter what, you won't always immediately understand why you feel the way you do; but if I remember the cycle, life happens → think → feel → act, you'll always have a framework for figuring a way forward.

If, on the other hand, you believe that everything happening outside of yourself creates how you feel, then you're going to end up spending an awful lot of time trying to control the outside world. You're going to get everything outside of you to line up just perfectly so that you can be happy. At some point, you'll discover that controlling the outside world is actually very hard to do; try as you might you just can't control everything. At that point, if you still feel bad, you're going to look for ways to distract yourself, and if you use alcohol as a crutch you're likely to turn to having a drink. You may have even found yourself in this situation before: "I don't know how to stop feeling anxious, unhappy, or lonely and I can't stand it" or "I don't even know what I'm feeling. I just know that something doesn't feel right, and I don't want to feel this way." Enter alcohol.

But when you realize that your thoughts create your emotions, you can turn your attention to the one thing you do have control over—your thinking.. This doesn't mean that you can change your thoughts by snapping your fingers. It will take practice. But it does mean that you have a way forward that doesn't involve dulling how you feel.

Let's go back to Claudia's story:

I feel so stupid. I spent the last year and a half putting my life on hold and trying to be the best girlfriend I could be to prove that he should care about me. I ignored all the signs telling me that this guy was not ready or interested in a relationship. As soon as I started drinking, I knew I couldn't keep it in anymore. I had to tell him how I really felt. Of course, he reacted terribly and we got in a huge drunken fight. He said he doesn't think we work together. If I hadn't gotten drunk and had just kept my mouth shut, none of this would have happened. I'm such an idiot.

Even if she knows how the cycle works, it's going to be difficult, if not impossible, to jump from the paragraph above to thinking: "It's all good, I'm better off anyway." But if she doesn't know how to change how she feels and has made a habit of using alcohol to feel better and numb feeling lonely, then after a break-up she's likely to dial up her drinking.

Many people have the experience of going back and forth between trying to control their environment and numbing their emotions in order to feel better. We chase after a relationship because we think that will make us happy, or we distract ourselves from our loneliness by having a drink. When we do find a partner, after the love-struck phase wears off, we'll wonder, "Why do I still feel empty on the inside?" and we'll go back to finding ways to distract ourselves from how we're feeling. Throughout all of this, we've ceded responsibility to everything outside of ourselves to make us feel better and change how we feel instead of realizing the incredible power we have to do this work from within. But we can't start that process until we learn how to sit with all our emotions instead of running from them.

Sitting with Your Emotions

Knowing that you can handle any emotion without using alcohol to numb how you're feeling is the amazing benefit of this work. Most people have a low tolerance for sitting with negative emotions. We become expert at pushing our emotions away, distracting ourselves, and, if we use alcohol as a crutch, numbing how we feel. But when we shift our focus to the physical manifestations that an emotion creates, we realize that we can tolerate whatever we are feeling in our body. The more familiar you are with the physical manifestations that accompany every emotion, the more you realize that you don't need to run away from sweaty palms, a clenched jaw, or a racing pulse. You are more than capable of learning how to sit with an emotion without covering up how you're feeling with a drink.

When you make a habit of resisting your negative emotions either by distracting yourself or numbing, you miss the unique physical sensations that coincide with each emotion. You may be so good at *not* feeling that, unless an emotion is very intense, you have a hard time identifying how you feel at all. You might think, "But I feel stressed/frustrated/anxious all the time—I want to feel this way less, not more!" But if you're really sitting with this emotion, if you're really open to fully experiencing it, can you articulate why exactly the physical manifestations of a negative emotion are so unbearable that you'll do anything to avoid it?

No emotional state can last forever. The physical changes to your body—the tingling, sweating, flushing, tensing, racing, etc.—cannot go on indefinitely. They will subside. When someone says she feels lonely or anxious or bored all the time, what she fails to realize is that she is thinking the thoughts that are creating these emotions over and over again, usually because she isn't even aware of the thoughts that are creating her feelings. The negative emotion is being created (and often reinforced) every time the thought comes up. Let's say you've been practicing awareness around your thoughts and notice that you're thinking the thought "I'm such a screw up" all the time. Each time you think it, you're producing the emotion of shame in your body. If you think the thought repeatedly, you'll repeatedly create shame. When you practice sitting with your emotions, you're effectively pausing the cycle and watching shame unfold in your body instead of reacting to how shame feels.

When people practice numbing how they feel, they never give themselves the opportunity to watch this happen. Instead, they quickly cover up how they are feeling. Not only that, refusing to let themselves experience an emotion doesn't make it go away. You know this already because we talk about "pushing our feelings down," "burying our emotions," or "holding everything in." All of these metaphors point us in the same direction: emotions want to be expressed. Most of us haven't learned to feel an emotion all the way through and let it run its course.

So many people are expert at resisting their emotions. Indeed, many of my clients are worried that their emotions might "take them over" or that if they let themselves fully feel a certain way they "won't be able to close the floodgates." Why do so many people have such resistance to feeling how they feel? I think it often goes back to what we learned (or didn't learn) as children. If no one teaches you what an emotion is or how it affects your body when you're little, the physical manifestations of a negative emotion can be frightening. You have no idea what is happening to you or why you feel the way you do. We aren't told that nothing has gone wrong, that our changes in our body are normal, or that while it may feel uncomfortable, an emotion can't hurt us. In fact, many people have the opposite experience. Growing up, they were specifically told to hold in how they were feeling, or they saw the adults around them struggling with their own emotions and modeled their behavior accordingly.

Here's how it works with drinking. My client, Alicia, wanted to stop feeling reliant on alcohol in social situations. When she socialized in big groups, she always felt uncomfortable and out of her element. She found herself totally caught up in her head and unable to enjoy herself. Having a couple of drinks loosened her up. She relaxed and became more talkative. The problem was that her job required a lot of post-work socializing, and she didn't like getting so tipsy, sometimes even drunk, in a professional setting.

Alicia tried to cut back, but her efforts were hit or miss. She tried cutting out alcohol altogether at these events, but she always found herself miserable and even started avoiding them. If she did go, Alicia would excuse herself at the first opportunity. Only then would she start to feel better. Alicia felt stuck. She didn't like the fact that she used alcohol as a crutch, worrying that if she drank too much she might overdo it, or that the only solution was to avoid going altogether.

When Alicia came to me, she knew she was feeling anxiety in these settings. She felt it all the time. What she really wanted was to figure out how to make her anxiety go away. But before we could work on changing how she was feeling, she had to start practicing staying with the physical manifestations of anxiety that made her so uncomfortable she wanted to either have a glass of wine or get the hell out of there.

Then Alicia started to get specific about how anxiety felt in her body. She noticed a queasy feeling in her stomach that was akin to a twisting—like her intestines were knotting up. She also realized that her muscles would tense up. Once she paid close attention, she noticed that her jaw and her hands were clenched the tightest. She even found herself grip her purse or a glass as if she was hanging on for dear life. Alicia started to understand more specifically how anxiety manifested in her body.

Instead of distracting herself or trying to change how she was feeling, Alicia started practicing paying attention to and watching these physical manifestations. She didn't have a drink to mask them, but she also didn't look for the first opportunity to remove herself from the situation. Alicia paid close attention to what was happening in her body. When she felt like she couldn't take it anymore, she would practice saying to herself, "This is what anxiety feels like in my body, and I can handle it." She soon discovered that while she didn't like these physical manifestations, they were, with practice, tolerable. She could handle them on her own. Soon she discovered something even more important: if she noticed the thoughts creating her anxiety and stayed with the awareness of what was happening in her body long enough, eventually it would subside.

This is the work of identifying, describing, and sitting with your emotions. Before you can start moving to feeling new, different emotions, you must be willing to be fully present with the ones you are running from. Once you become an expert at identifying the physical manifestations associated with your negative emotions, you'll find yourself less likely to push them away or cover them up with a drink.

Keep in mind that the way an emotion feels is different for every person. Sadness for me feels like my body is constricting. My chest tightens, making it difficult to take a full breath. I feel my throat closing up. My shoulders start to slump, my stomach pulls in, and I can feel my body wanting to curl up into a ball. If the feeling is particularly intense, I'll notice almost a buzzing in my chest cavity. Crying starts first in my nose as a tingling sensation that moves toward my eyes. For as long as I can remember, I fought with all my might to stop myself from ever feeling sad. If I felt like I was going to cry, I did everything possible to push the feeling away. Observing the emotion, gave me more authority over it. I no longer needed to run from how I felt.

You can't snap your fingers and start feeling something different. If you're used to viewing your emotions as something that you need to cover up and hide from, you must first learn that every emotion is tolerable. You do this by paying attention to the physical manifestations. Only then, when you see that your emotions can't really harm you, and that you don't need to be afraid of them, can you really learn that you don't need to use alcohol as the way out. Only then can you begin the process of moving to a new and better feeling emotion (more on this in Chapter 8).

Exercise 4: Observing Your Emotions
Time Required: 10 minutes

Emotions are one-word feeling states—happy, angry, sad, nervous— that physically manifest in your body. Depending on the emotion you are feeling, your breathing slows down or speeds up, your muscles tense or relax, and different parts of your body flush or feel cold, etc. The only way to learn that all your emotions are tolerable is to get familiar with these signs and know that you can withstand them.

A body scan is the best way to identify and describe the physical manifestations of an emotion. You can use this exercise in two different ways:

- **Set aside time each day to practice the body scan**: When you first start out, you'll want to make time for regular practice so that you can familiarize yourself with the tool. You can do this at any point in the day, but some people find a body scan is particularly helpful in the afternoon or evening when their negative emotions seem the strongest.
- **Use the tool whenever you feel a particularly strong emotion**: When your emotions are loud, the physical manifestations are the most noticeable. Try using this tool if you just lost your temper, burst into tears, or are feeling very impatient.

Follow these steps (Read all the way through the instructions before you begin):

- **Find a comfortable place to sit down, set a timer for five minutes, and close your eyes.**
- **Start, by bringing you attention to your feet.** Feel your feet pressed into the floor. Notice your connection to the ground.
- **Slowly move your attention through the different parts of your body until you reach the crown of your head.** As you work your way up, see if you notice any physical changes (e.g., tension, flushing, sweating, shaking, heart racing). Pay particular attention to your jaw, hands, forehead, shoulders, back and neck. Is your breathing regular, shallow, fast or slow, or are you holding your breath?

- **If you finish before the five minutes are up, go back and start from your feet.** Keep scanning your body until the timer goes off.

Spend the next five minutes jotting down what you noticed:

- **What emotion do you think you are experiencing?** *Remember, emotions are a single word: glad, sad, mad, etc. "I feel terrible" is a thought, not an emotion. If you're not sure what emotion you are experiencing, take a guess. There's no right or wrong answer. You'll get better at identifying different emotions the more you practice.*
- **How is this emotion manifesting in my body?** *Did you notice things like tension, flushing, sweating, shaking, or heart racing?*
- **Where is this emotion located in my body?** *Did you notice that specific areas were affected (e.g., your jaw, hands, forehead, shoulders, back and neck?). Did the sensation stay in one place or move around?*
- **Are the physical effects of this emotion tolerable?** *Are the sensations you described something you think you can tolerate? Why or why not?*
- **Why am I feeling this emotion?** *Write down the reason why you think you're experiencing this emotion. Remember, you never feel an emotion until you think a thought.*

Once you get good at using a body scan you can use it wherever you are. You don't need to sit down or close your eyes. You just need to tune into and observe what is happening in your body.

5   The Role of Your Urges

The Pull to Drink

When my clients start working with these tools, one of the most frustrating steps is often dealing with the urge to drink. They're starting to get the hang of the think → feel → act cycle and at times can even watch it in action. They're learning how to identify and sit with uncomfortable emotions. But then, without warning, the pull to drink rears its head. Sometimes, it comes on so strong and so suddenly that they worry they're doing something wrong. Worse, they worry that their desire to drink is a sign that they may never figure out how to stop using alcohol as a crutch.

Remember back in Chapter 2 when I talked about habits and how they are created through repetition? Well repetition isn't the only component necessary for creating a habit. Your brain also needs a cue and a reward. The cue is a sign to your brain that it should begin activating the habit, and the reward reinforces the habit by letting your brain know that there's a benefit waiting on the other side. It works this way with all habits, not just drinking. Repeat the pattern enough and one day you'll find yourself walking through the door after a long day of work and start to open a bottle of wine without even thinking about it. Coming home was your brain's cue to activate the habit, and your brain is already looking forward to the reward waiting at the bottom of a glass.

Just because you've taught yourself a habit doesn't mean you don't have control or free will. You are not doomed to follow habits blindly. But keep in mind, the whole point of having habits is so that your brain can be its most efficient by moving patterns into your unconscious. Your brain cares only about saving energy, and habits help it do just that by automating an action. Your brain doesn't discriminate between "good" and "bad" habits. It just wants to be as efficient as possible. If you have a habit running in the background (for example, using alcohol as a crutch), the way to change it is to bring awareness to the think → feel → act cycle so that you can figure out what is driving the habit and pinpoint how to change it.

Needs vs. Wants

Every habit needs a cue, a sign to start the habit. A cue can be anything—a time of day, an event, an emotion, a smell, a particular food, an object, a sound, or even certain people. Once you encounter the cue, an urge bubbles up. Most of us aren't tuned into our cues, and so it can feel like our urges come from out of nowhere. That's never the case because all of our habits have cues.

Here's the tricky part: once you recognize your cues, most people assume that these cues *cause* their urges (the same way people assume that their external environment creates their feelings). You know from the think → feel → act cycle that this isn't the case. Your actions are always driven by your emotions, which were in turn created by your thoughts. You never take an action without feeling an emotion first, and your emotions are always created by a thought. You may have specific thoughts that you think when you see a cue, but the thought, not the cue itself, creates the urge to drink.

The trouble is that once we've developed a habit, the think → feel → act cycle has moved into our unconscious, so it feels as though there isn't a thought. You're not yet aware of what you're thinking. Here's the good news: an urge is just the emotion of desire. It's created by the think → feel → act cycle. Better still, you already have experience at managing your desires. After all, having a drink is not the only desire you've ever had. You desire things all the time. Maybe you desire chocolate or a new wardrobe or a vacation. You already have practice managing lots of desires without even realizing it.

Before going into more about desire, you need to understand the difference between a need and a want. There are things that your body *needs* to have in order to function. Your needs are driven by your impulse to survive. They include things like:

- Oxygen
- Water
- Food
- Sleep
- Warmth

Your body is driven to survive and seek the things that it *truly* needs to function. You can't, for example, hold your breath indefinitely or decide that you no longer need sleep. Your needs are for the most part truly outside of your control. When it comes to your needs, your body requires a basic level of each so that it can function and maintain homeostasis. Your needs aren't part of the think → feel → act cycle.

It is possible your body can become physically dependent on alcohol (i.e., your body becomes physically ill without the substance). Most people who want to change their relationship with alcohol are nowhere near the point of suffering tremors, shakiness, or sweating when they aren't drinking. If you cannot function without alcohol or think that you have become physically dependent or addicted, you should seek medical attention.

Your wants are different from your needs. Your wants are not necessary for survival, even though they sometimes feel like they are. When alcohol becomes a crutch, you *think* you need it in order to feel better or make a situation more bearable. But, of course, you don't really need it. You've just taught your brain that it makes a situation easier, and you've practiced using it so often that it has become a habit that you don't know how to unravel. In reality, you aren't practiced sitting with discomfort.

The biological urges to eat, sleep, breathe, and keep ourselves warm that control your survival are not the same as your desire. Your desires are connected to your thoughts. You desire things because you believe they will help you feel a certain way.

Understanding Pleasure

There are, of course, stimuli in your external environment that can induce temporary physical pleasure, much like there are things in your environment that can create physical pain. Having a glass of wine, eating a piece of chocolate, or getting a massage can all create the sensation of pleasure just as stubbing your toe or biting your tongue creates the sensation of pain. As with your emotions, pleasure and physical pain create different sensations in your body. The key difference is the point of origin. Pleasure and physical pain start in your body—you drink something, eat something, or something touches you—and the sensation travels from the point of origin to your mind. Emotions work in reverse.

Because your emotions are created by your thoughts, an emotion will start in your mind and travel to your body.

You probably aren't used to making these distinctions, but especially when you're trying to stop using alcohol as a crutch it's important to differentiate between the two. The emotion of happiness that you create with your thoughts is not the same as the pleasure you get when you have a drink. First, the buzz from alcohol always wears off—it is only sustained as long as you keep ingesting the substance (most people notice the initial pleasure from alcohol decreases with each drink). Second, it's possible to develop a tolerance to alcohol so it takes more to achieve the same result. Finally, the pleasurable effect of alcohol comes with a cost. You might wake up the next day feeling groggy, nauseous, headachy, or just blue for no reason. The same cannot be said for the emotion of happiness.

Because we aren't taught the think → feel → act cycle, we go about trying to feel good by external means—finding things in our external environment that can create the feeling of pleasure. This sensation is only ever temporary. You know this already: a massage may make you feel relaxed, but the relaxation you get can't sustain you through a stressful week. Eating chocolate is enjoyable, but that enjoyment is fleeting and doesn't last much beyond the moment you consume it. And alcohol can give you a buzz, but once the buzz has worn off so too has the pleasure.

Don't get me wrong, I'm not suggesting that the goal is to live life as an ascetic and swear off all forms of pleasure. Pleasure is an essential part of life, and I would never choose to experience life without it. But relying on external things that create pleasure as your *primary* way to feel good is not only unsustainable but usually brings with it a new set of problems. Drink too much and you'll have a hangover. Eat too much and you'll gain weight. Spend too much and you won't be able to pay your credit card bills. On the other hand, if you use the think → feel → act cycle you'll find that it is accessible in any moment, without bringing a new set of problems. Yes, it takes practice and effort. It isn't a quick and easy fix like pouring a glass of wine or having a bowl of ice cream, but the results are much more long lasting and have positive consequences.

React, Resist, Distract, Observe

Back to urges. Remember an urge is just the emotion of desire. The object of an urge is not something your body needs to survive; it is something you want to have because you think it will make you feel a certain way. Just asking yourself the simple question, "Is this something I *need* to survive or something that I *want* to have?" can start to give you clarity about what's really going on. Once you understand that your desire for something is created by your thoughts you can begin to have authority over your desire.

My clients will sometimes tell me that an urge can feel impossible to resist or that they just had to give in. Think back to Chapter 4 on understanding your emotions. There you learned how to sit with and observe an emotion. Of course, observing is not the only response you can have. When it comes to your emotions, you can also react, resist, and distract. Let's take a look at the emotions of anger and sadness to understand the different responses before delving into the desire to drink. Keep in mind that the ways in which you react, resist, distract, and observe your emotions are unique to you and may not fit with the following descriptions:

ANGER
- <u>React</u>: *You lose your temper, snap at someone, throw a pillow, or stomp your foot.*
- <u>Resist</u>: *You sit very still, arms crossed, lips pursed with smoke coming out of your ears.*
- <u>Distract</u>: *You turn on the TV, go shopping, or pour yourself a drink—anything to help you forget how you're feeling.*

- Observe: *You sit down, take a deep breath, and pay attention to how anger feels in your body. You notice your heart is racing, your back muscles are tense, and your jaw is clenched. You don't try to make this go away. You allow yourself to watch how anger feels in your body knowing that it will eventually pass.*

SADNESS

- React: *You're sobbing and your chest heaves as you gasp for air. You're completely overwhelmed by your thoughts and are sure this feeling will never go away.*
- Resist: *You fight back tears and try to stop your chin from quivering. You tell yourself you aren't allowed to cry.*
- Distract: *You're too busy to be sad, so you put a smile on your face and make yourself so busy you don't have a moment to think about how you feel.*
- Observe: *You feel sadness coming on and allow it to wash over you. You feel a slight buzzing sensation start in your chest that seems almost as if it is moving. Tears stream down your face, and you notice the saltiness in your tears. You are allowing yourself to be sad and aren't scared that you will be consumed by this emotion.*

Does any of this sound familiar? Do you have a sense of the different ways in which you react, resist, and distract from your emotions? The same thing happens when you have an urge to drink. In that moment, you can choose to react, resist, distract, or observe the desire inside of you.

THE URGE TO DRINK

- React: *You buy a bottle of wine and pour yourself a glass or you head to the bar and order a drink.*

- Resist: *You use all your willpower to say no over and over again. Your body feels tense and constricted and your breathing is shallow. You feel like you're fighting yourself and may notice that you start fidgeting or wanting to move your hands or your feet. You feel like you are white-knuckling it through your desire.*
- Distract: *You remove yourself from the situation where people are drinking. You turn on the TV. You eat something sweet. Anything to keep yourself busy so you don't have to be face-to-face with your urge.*
- Observe: *You feel the urge in your body. You notice a singular focus in your mind and the sensation of rushing. You take a couple of deep breaths. You're not afraid of the urge because you know if you sit with it long enough and stay present the urge will eventually go away on its own. You know that you are not at its mercy—you always have free will.*

The question is this: Why does the desire to drink feel so strong and why are urges to drink so intense? If you use alcohol as a crutch to escape discomfort, then two things have happened: First, you're very practiced at saying yes to a drink (i.e., reacting) when your desire appears, in which case you've taught your brain there is a strong pleasure reward associated with saying yes. Second, you've unconsciously taught yourself that you can dull specific negative emotions, which is a kind of reward in and of itself.

Essentially, your brain is very used to getting *two* rewards whenever you say yes to an urge and have a drink. Go back and look at what happens when you react to anger or sadness. There isn't the same reward structure built into these reactions. The urge to drink feels so intense because you've taught your brain there is a greater reward for reacting. You've conditioned your brain to expect a reward whenever the desire to drink arises. Every time you said yes, the habit was strengthened.

Think back to how habits work: your brain wants the think → feel → act cycle to be unconscious. Because you never understood how your desire was created, it seems as if the pull alcohol has on you materializes out of nowhere.

Habits are challenging to replace because we don't understand how they work. They can be so mysterious that at times it feels like we are acting against our own will, for example, when we drink more than we intended. By observing an urge, you are working to bring this habit back to your full consciousness and uncover the thoughts creating your desire. Nothing is wrong with you because you feel an urge. It's exactly how your brain is supposed to work.

What an Urge Feels Like

Understanding what an urge feels like in your body is crucial to this process. Right now, you may not have the vocabulary to describe what an urge feels like in your body. That's okay. Most likely it's because you're very practiced at reacting to the urge to drink (i.e., pouring yourself a glass). You may be so practiced that it feels as if there isn't any time between the desire to drink arising and your reaction.

How many times have you felt like you didn't make a conscious decision to pour yourself another glass of wine; it just happened? The feeling of not actively deciding makes perfect sense when you think about how habits work in the brain. You don't think; you just do. This doesn't just happen with drinking—it happens in all sorts of areas in your life.

Remember, repetition is necessary for learning. You repeat the think → feel → act cycle enough that the habit becomes unconscious. When you get behind a wheel of a car you don't have to think of the hundreds of steps involved in pulling out of a driveway. You just get in and go. If you drive a regular route to work each day, you've probably had the experience of arriving home from work and feeling like you barely remember the drive. Your habit took over while your brain wandered.

Without understanding how habits are formed and the think → feel → act cycle, pouring yourself a glass without even realizing it can be scary. It feels as if you're not fully in control, and most people don't like that feeling. But just because your brain is executing a habit does not mean that you are not in control or that you'll be unable to bring consciousness to it. All it means is that you must make a deliberate practice of being aware. You must bring back mindfulness to your actions.

The good news is that drinking is not the only place in your life where you experience urges or where you've developed habits. This means that you can start paying attention to what urges feel like in other areas of your life, not just drinking. Here are just a few:

- Eating (especially any foods that you find hard to resist or the pace at which you eat)
- Checking your phone (think of how often you reach for it without even thinking)
- Social media (one moment you're writing in Word and the next Facebook is open)

You can also bring attention to anything you do on autopilot. Walking is a great example. Unless you have an injury, you probably don't pay attention to your gait even though it's an extremely complicated movement that requires different levels of coordinated activity. There's so much to notice. The part of your feet that hits the ground first, the distribution of your weight (forward or back), the rotation of your knees, the tilt of your pelvis, the direction of your spine, the placement of your shoulders, the swing of your arms, and the position of your head. All of these things will help you build the skill of mindfulness and awareness that will help unravel your habit of using alcohol as a crutch.

As for urges, you'll notice that they have one thing in common: they feel fast. There is a speed to them. There's a quickness to the action. Noticing how this pace feels in your body is crucial. Strong urges usually have an insistence and an urgency behind them. A sensation of *now*. Bringing mindfulness to this moment is how you work to slow the urge down so you can begin the process of unwinding it.

Exercise 5: Observing Your Urges

Time Required: Allow as much time as needed

Urges cannot last forever. Sometimes this fact alone is reassuring. Like emotions, they will eventually pass. Most of us are practiced at doing something in response to an urge (and not just the urge to drink). We have the feeling that an urge *must* be dealt with right away. It *must* be tended to. When we're trying to change a habit, the very presence of an urge can make people feel like they're doing something wrong.

It's easy to assume that if I want to change something that isn't serving me I shouldn't desire to do it anymore. That your logic should supersede habit (i.e., if I don't want to drink, I should no longer desire it.). But that's not how habits work. Too often, people assume that the presence of an urge means something is wrong. Nothing is wrong. Even when you have practice under your belt, urges may continue to appear. The trick is not to make your urges mean anything about you or your progress. The best way to be able to do this is to practice observing an urge. Letting it in, watching it, and not being afraid of its presence.

There's nothing wrong with resisting or distracting yourself from an urge—especially in the beginning. But resisting and distracting are not very good long-term solutions. If you rely only on willpower, at some point you'll probably find yourself exhausted and may not have the energy to say no. If you focus on removing all temptation, when someone offers you a drink (and trust me they will) you won't have practiced what to do in the moment when faced with an urge. In fact, you need to experience urges so that you can start the process of bringing consciousness to your habit and the thoughts driving the think → feel → act cycle. It's a good thing when urges arise because it gives you a window into your mind. Working on observing your urges is the best way to get some authority in the moment.

After a while, your urges will lessen as you start to see how the think → feel → act cycle creates your desire. In this moment it's easy to fool yourself into thinking you've worked at this long enough that you should be free of urges from here on out. Think about it this way; how many times did you say yes to your desire to drink? For me, the number was surely in the thousands. There was nothing wrong if an urge appeared after a long period of not having any. It only mattered if I made it mean something negative about me or my progress.

Most people I work with struggle at first to understand if they're observing an urge or resisting it. It's easier to tell when you are reacting (pouring yourself a drink) or distracting (occupying your mind elsewhere). At first, the difference between resisting and observing can be harder to parse. The biggest clue is to pay attention to any tension in your body and the depth of your breathing. If you feel clenched and taking shallow breaths, you're most likely resisting.

Because an urge is just the emotion of desire, you'll notice the technique here is similar to Exercise 4: Observing Your Emotions. Practicing this skill on your own is ideal, but not always realistic, because urges may arise when you're out with other people. Do your best to practice the skill wherever you are.

Follow these steps when an urge arises (set aside as much time as needed):

- **First, take several slow, deep breaths.** When an urge arises, we tend to hold our breath. You want to keep breathing as much as possible.
- **Remind yourself that urges are normal.** Nothing has gone wrong. Feeling an urge doesn't mean that your habit is getting stronger or that it will be impossible to break. Every urge will eventually pass if you stay present with it.
- **Notice if there is any tension in your body.** Pay particular attention to your jaw, hands, forehead, shoulders, back and neck. If you find an area of tension, move your focus there and take a deep breath.
- **See if you can notice where in your body the urge resides.** Scan your body from your feet to the crown of your head. Be on the lookout for any physical changes (e.g., tension, flushing, sweating, shaking, heart racing).
- **Pay attention to any thoughts that come up.** What thoughts run through your mind when you are trying to observe the urge?
- **Keep breathing.** The urge will subside if you are open to observing. See if you can notice the urge peak and then taper off. You might notice that the urge seems to come in waves. This is perfectly normal, and is nothing to worry about. It's just your habit on repeat.

As soon as possible, answer the following questions:

- **How did the urge manifest in your body?** Did you notice that specific areas were affected (e.g., your jaw, hands, forehead, shoulders, back and neck?) Were there any physical sensations (e.g., shallow breathing, tension, flushing, sweating, shaking, heart racing)?

- **Do you think you were resisting or observing the urge?**
  Were you able to breathe normally or did your breathing feel
  shallow or constrained? Did parts of your body feel tense, tight,
  restricted or constricted?
- **Are the physical effects of the urge tolerable?** Are these
  sensations you described something you think you can tolerate.
  Why or why not?
- **What thoughts came up for you while you were observing
  the urge?** It's common to have thoughts about the efficacy of
  the exercise, the time it is taking for an urge to pass, your ability
  to see this through, or reasons why you should just give in.
  What came up for you?
- **Why do you think you experienced the urge?** There's no right
  or wrong answer. Once you start keeping regular track of your
  urges, you'll begin to notice patterns and the cues associated
  with the habit. Pay particular attention to specific times of day,
  emotions, events, or people.

You'll want to keep track of your urges so that you can see the
progress you've made. Chapter 6 will show you how to record your urges.
Noticing and observing an urge, instead of reacting, takes practice. Don't
expect to be perfect at it or never give in. This is a process. If you decide
to drink, nothing has gone wrong. In fact, there's a wealth of valuable
information for you in that moment to understand better your think →
feel → act cycle.

Unwinding Your Desire to Drink

Now that you understand that an urge is just the emotion of desire and
how important it is to be able to observe an urge instead of reacting,
resisting, or distracting, it's useful to go deeper and learn to see how our
thinking creates our desires.

The think → feel → act cycle is at play whenever an urge arises. Your urges are connected to cues: urges come at a certain time of day, specific situations or at particular events. Recognizing and anticipating your cues will help you get better at working with your urges. When you know an urge is likely to arise, you can prepare for it and plan how to handle your desire to drink. Just remember that, specific times of day, situations, people, and events do not create your desire to drink. Just like everything else in the think → feel → act cycle, we always think a thought before we experience an emotion. The same is true with the urge (i.e., the emotion of desire) to drink. In this case, you've unconsciously connected a specific thought to a cue. Because the cycle has been repeated so many times and the habit is unconscious we mistakenly believe the cycle works like this: cue → feel → act. For example:

- *get home from work → feel the urge to drink → have a drink*
- *dinner with friends → feel the urge to drink → have a drink*
- *happy hour with co-workers → feel the urge to drink → have a drink*

As you already know, the cycle doesn't work this way. Your external environment is not the cause of your emotions—or your desire to drink—your thoughts are. If you're going to unwind an urge, you need to first identify the thoughts creating the desire. There are lots of them, but here's a small sample:

- I deserve a drink.
- Just this once.
- One glass won't hurt.
- This is so unfair.
- I need a drink.
- I just need a break.

- I really want a drink.
- I need to relax.
- I want to join in.
- This is no fun without alcohol.
- It doesn't matter.
- This is too hard.
- Screw this.
- F*** it.
- I want to.
- I hate having to say no.
- I feel so uncomfortable right now.

For most of us, the thought that triggers our desire is so automatic and so unconscious that we don't even notice it. But once we pay attention, we start to understand how the cycle really works: cue → *think* → feel → act. For example:

- get home from work → "I just need a break." → feel the urge to drink → have a drink
- dinner with friends → "I want to join in." → feel the urge to drink → have a drink
- happy hour with co-workers → "This is boring without alcohol." → feel the urge to drink → have a drink

If you want to unwind your desire to drink, you have to identify the thought that is creating it.

Part of what is confusing is the common belief that if someone has stopped drinking it is extremely difficult to be around alcohol. People will occasionally ask me if it's okay for them to drink in front of me. The idea that people who struggle with alcohol can't control themselves is connected, not only to the idea of being powerless, but also to the idea that our urges are created by our cues. In many ways, this belief makes sense because we're conditioned to believe that all emotions—including desire—are created by our external environment.

Especially when you're getting started, there's absolutely no problem with taking yourself out of environments where you experience a lot of urges. But it's important to remember that the environments themselves are not creating the urges—it's always your thinking about that environment. When I teach this to my clients, it usually comes as a huge relief. It means you don't have to sequester yourself so that you avoid alcohol at all costs. You don't need to limit your socializing to completely dry settings where no one is drinking, nor do you need to ask your friends, your family, and your romantic partner to stop drinking in front of you. In fact, once you get some practice observing your urges (as opposed to reacting to them) being around alcohol can be really useful as an opportunity to notice your thoughts about it. Once you have this insight, you can see what's creating your urges and practice new thoughts that will help unwind your desire.

I've said this earlier, but it is worth repeating: the think → feel → act cycle is also why I believe it's possible to get to a place where you don't desire to drink. If alcohol is the thing creating your desire, you're pretty much stuck. Alcohol has been with us for thousands of years, and it isn't going anywhere anytime soon. On the other hand, if your thoughts create your desire, you're in luck. From this position, you can observe, change, practice, and eventually develop new automatic thoughts associated with drinking.

On my own journey, one of the most important thoughts that I identified that created my desire to drink was "I just want to be normal." It might seem innocuous, but for me this thought was toxic. When I thought, "I just want to be normal," I wanted to be like everyone else, and to me that meant drinking. I was able to exert willpower, but after a while it got to be too much. The problem was that the thought "I just want to be normal" was still there and kept perpetuating my desire.

I learned how to start slowly changing the thought, "I just want to be normal." It was a thought I had a lot of practice thinking, so it certainly didn't change overnight. Once I started to unpack what was fueling it, namely a narrative that people in our society who struggle with alcohol have a character defect, I began to be able to chip away at it. For me, this has been a much more sustainable and in the long-run an easier process. Instead of focusing on saying no over and over again, I was able break the think → feel → act cycle that was creating my desire to drink in the first place. Eventually, I no longer had to resist my desire because my thoughts weren't creating it.

Exercise 6: The Thoughts That Fuel Your Desire

Time Required: 30 minutes

An urge is just the emotion of desire. Now that you understand how it figures into the think → feel → act → cycle, you have a framework for understanding how to begin to unwind it. If your thoughts create your emotions, then you need to identify the thought creating your desire.

Exercise 5: Observing Your Urges, should have given you some insight into your thinking around urges. This exercise will take your insight to the next step and pinpoint the thoughts that fuel your desire. You can use this exercise in two different ways:

- **Option A: Record what you're thinking in the moment when the urge to drink arises**: Once you have some practice under your belt observing your urges, you can move to recording what you're thinking when your desire arises.
- **Option B: Investigate the thinking you have around specific situations that usually involve the urge to drink**: Make a list

of all the cues in which you feel the urge to drink (when I get home from work, dinner with friends, when I'm at a bar, when I can't fall asleep, the holidays, a wedding, etc.). You'll use this exercise to uncover the thoughts you have about drinking in each of these situations.

Follow these steps:

- **Set a timer for two minutes, and grab a sheet of paper.**
- **Option A: On a piece of paper write down everything that you're thinking during the urge**. Remember you aren't journaling. You're trying to capture your stream of consciousness. Don't edit yourself.
- **Option B: Select one situation from your list. Write it at the top of your paper.** Write down all the thinking that comes up when you think about not drinking in this situation. Same as Option A, don't edit yourself.
- **Keep your pen moving.** Don't think about what you "should" write; just write. If nothing comes up, just keep writing, "I don't know what I'm thinking" over and over again. Your thoughts will eventually surface if you keep your pen moving.
- **As you write down your thoughts, try to be curious rather than judgmental.** The temptation is always to start judging what you're thinking and then start editing. Pay attention to any thoughts you resist putting on paper.

Once the two minutes is up, spend the remaining time examining what you wrote.

- **Underline any thoughts that stand out to you or feel particularly strong:** You'll probably have lots of thoughts that come up, but some will feel familiar (i.e., you realize you think this all the time) or will produce a strong gut reaction. If you're not sure, just pick one from what you wrote. There's no right or wrong way to do this.

- **Select one thought that you'd like to practice changing**: Of the thoughts that you underlined, select one thought that you'd like to practice changing.
- **Brainstorm at least five alternatives for this thought**: Not all thoughts are the same. You need to select something that feels believable and motivating to you. Remember, you can't move from "This is impossible" to "This is easy" overnight. You need to find a more neutral option like "I am capable of practicing these tools." The more you brainstorm, the better chance of coming up with something that will work for you.

Here are some sample thoughts that may fuel your desire to drink and neutral alternatives to get you started.

Desire-Fueling Thoughts	Neutral Thought Alternatives
I deserve a drink.	I want to show myself I can do this.
Just this once.	I am stronger than this urge.
One glass won't hurt.	An urge can't hurt me.
This is so unfair.	I'm learning something by sitting with the urge.
I want to.	This is just a habit that I can unlearn.
I need a drink.	I want a drink, but I don't need a drink.
I just need a break.	There are other ways to give myself a break.

I really want a drink.	I can make it through this without a drink.
I need to relax.	I need to take a deep breath.
I want to join in.	I can join in without drinking.
This is no fun without alcohol.	I can figure out ways to make this fun.
It doesn't matter.	Every time I observe an urge, it matters.
This is too hard.	I am strong enough to do this.
Screw this.	An urge will always pass.
F*** it.	Whatever is bothering me I can handle.
I hate having to say no.	I am saying yes to me.
I feel so uncomfortable.	I can handle discomfort.

- **Select one thought you can see yourself practicing**: Write this thought down on a post-it note and carry it around with you or make it a reminder on your phone. Recite the thought in the morning and again when you experience an urge or before you head into a situation where you would typically drink (e.g., coming home at the end of the day or meeting friends at a bar). Try it out for a week and see if it helps relieve some of your desire. If not, try a new thought.

The work of changing your thoughts can seem tedious at first, but remember that you've been practicing the thoughts that create your desire to drink for a very long time. Ultimately, you'll want to work through all the thoughts that you identify and find alternatives. Every week you can pick a new thought to work on and try out an alternative. With steady practice, you can change the think → feel → act → cycle and unwind your desire to drink.

How to Take a
Break from Drinking

There's Never a Good Time To Start

Have you ever thought about taking a break from drinking and told yourself, "Now just isn't a good time"?

- Things are too stressful at home. I need a break from everything.
- I should really wait until after vacation. Otherwise, my time away will be no fun.
- The wedding I have to attend next month is going to be unbearable if I stop now.
- I would, but dating without drinking is next to impossible.
- I'll start after the holidays. I have way too many events on my calendar.

You know what happens? You keep waiting and waiting for the "right" time to change, and sure enough the right time never appears. There's always something standing in your way. Why?

Until now, you've thought that your emotions were created by what's happening in your life, so you kept waiting for life to let up a little. I hope by now you are at least challenging that assumption. Think about the co-worker that never seems to get frazzled by crazy demands at work, the friend who doesn't lose her temper when she's stuck in traffic, or the person that stays calm under pressure and somehow rises to the challenge instead of crumbling.

We know these people exist. We know that not everyone reacts the same under the same circumstances. Yet we explain away these differences by declaring, "I'm just not built that way" or "This is just my personality," and we can go back to attributing how we feel to everything that's happening externally in our lives. Because of this, we stall. We know that change is going to be hard, so we think we should wait for everything outside of us to ease up. You don't need life to ease up; you need to find better-feeling thoughts.

You know from the preceding chapters that circumstances don't dictate how you feel; your thoughts do. You don't need to find the "right" time to change because there is no "right" time. The stars don't have to align and create the perfect set of circumstances. You can either begin now or you can wait.

Change is always challenging. It's supposed to be. You're learning a new way of doing things, and learning takes work. We have to practice over and over because the only way to hardwire a new habit is through repetition. You won't be able to handle your emotions better when everything in your life lines up perfectly; thank goodness because that will never happen. You'll be able to handle your emotions better when you realize what really causes them (your thoughts). Once you know what causes your emotions and how to change them using the think → feel → act → cycle, you won't need to rely on alcohol to feel better or to distract yourself from how you really feel. When deciding whether to take a break, you need to look at the situation from every angle and decide what's right for you. But before you do this, let's cover some of the most common fears about taking a break.

The Fears Holding You Back

Before creating your plan of action, I want to discuss the fears I see most often with my clients:

"I'm afraid that any plan I make isn't going to work because I've failed in the past." In all likelihood, this isn't your first attempt to reign in your drinking. You've made other plans in the past. Maybe you stuck to them for a while, but eventually you fell back into your old ways. Why should this time be any different? If you're anything like me, your previous plans probably focused on two things:

- How much you were drinking (either abstaining completely or setting limits).
- Using willpower to resist the urge to drink.

What you've learned in this book is different. All your energy is not focused on *how much* you're drinking or saying no by using willpower. Rather, I want you to understand what makes drinking so appealing in the first place and help you find new ways to give yourself those same benefits without alcohol (More on that in Chapter 8). The goal here is not to focus on using willpower and discipline to resist the urge to drink. Instead, you'll use the think → feel → act cycle to understand what is creating the urge and use this information to dismantle the urge from its source: your thoughts. At the very least, this will be a totally new approach for you.

"I think this is going to be too hard and change will be too difficult." Changing habits requires work, and yes, sometimes it will be hard, but it's by no means impossible. In the long run, attempting to break out of this habit is much faster than keeping with the status quo. You have two choices:

- Keep things as they are and hope that your struggle will magically resolve itself, or
- Start learning and practicing a new way forward

Here's where most people get tripped up. Because the process of changing habits is difficult, you are apt to make the difficulty you encounter mean something about who you are or your likelihood of succeeding. Don't fall for this trap. Don't tell yourself that because change is hard you'll never figure this out or that you're doing something wrong. When you think these thoughts the think → feel → act cycle springs to action. The thoughts "I'm never going to figure this out; I'm doing something wrong; or Change is impossible" make you feel hopeless. And when you feel hopeless, you're likely to give up before you get started.

The fact that changing a habit is difficult means absolutely nothing about you or your ability to succeed. The best way to think about this is to look at an example that has nothing to do with drinking and no cultural narratives connected to it: touch typing. Touch typing is using your muscle memory to find keys on a keyboard so that you can type while keeping your eyes on the screen. If you know how to touch type, you learned on a QWERTY keyboard (so named because the letters q, w, e, r, t, y run from left to right on the top letter row). If you've mastered touch typing, you can type with your eyes closed. You've practiced enough times that you don't need to think about where the correct keys are; your fingers just seem to know.

What do you think would happen if I gave you a completely new keyboard to type on? One that didn't use the QWERTY layout, but instead listed the letters in alphabetical order. The layout of an ABCDEF keyboard would make perfect sense. Intellectually you would understand how it works because it follows the alphabet. But just because you understand the how the ABCDEF keyboard works doesn't mean that you would be able to automatically touch type using it. Certainly, not on your first go, especially since your brain already has the QWERTY habit down pat. At first, if you needed to draft an email, you would probably have to hunt and peck in order to find the correct keys. Typing would be excruciatingly slow, but with effort and patience you would be able to finish.

Here's the thing, you would forever have to hunt and peck unless you purposefully tried to teach yourself to touch type using the ABCDEF keyboard. Even if you got really good at hunting and pecking, in the back of your mind you'd probably think, "I hate the ABCDEF keyboard. It's so slow. Everything was so much better and easier with the QWERTY keyboard." You would likely wish for the QWERTY keyboard and always think that the new one was inferior.

What if you committed yourself to learning to touch type on the new ABCDEF keyboard? Even if you were dedicated and set aside time to practice every day you would make mistakes. You'd get some steam going, and then one of your fingers would go for the wrong letter. Your brain would get tripped up and go back to the old QWERTY habit. Now you could tell yourself, "Screwing up means I'm doing this wrong" or you could remind yourself that, "It's impossible to unlearn a habit perfectly on the first try." Making mistakes is part of the process. It's how your brain learns to replace an old habit with a new one. You have to mess up in order to create the new neural pathways. Making a mistake means absolutely nothing about you. It doesn't mean that you're doing something wrong or that you'll never figure it out. It's just part of the learning process.

When things get hard, we tend to make it mean something about ourselves. Instead of seeing it as a necessary part of the process of learning, we tell ourselves it means something negative about who we are. This is especially true when you're trying to change a habit like your drinking, which is mired in stories like, "The world is divided into normal drinkers and alcoholics" or "Regular people don't struggle with their drinking." If you wouldn't make the struggle and the time required to learn a new keyboard mean something negative about who you are, then don't let the struggle to stop using alcohol as a crutch mean something negative about you either.

This is a terrible cycle to get stuck in. Whenever you're frustrated by the process or telling yourself that change is too hard, make sure you ask yourself, "What am I making this mean about me?" You need to make sure you're aware of the negative thought patterns that make you want to throw in the towel.

"I'm worried that I still feel ambivalent about wanting to change." For many people, just feeling ambivalent holds them back because they think that they need to feel 100 percent sure that taking a break is the right direction before they can get started.

I was also ambivalent when I started this process. I wasn't sure I really wanted to stop drinking, I wasn't sure that my life would actually turn out better or that I would ultimately be happier. I knew stopping would remove all the repercussions from drinking too much, but deep down I felt like I would always be on the outside looking in. I worried that by not drinking I would be missing out on life.

I had to give up on certainty as a necessary ingredient for moving forward. I didn't want to risk failure because I thought that failure would mean something about me. Ultimately, the only thing that I could be certain of was the effort I put in to change. That's it. I could make a commitment to show up, try something new, pick myself up when I stumbled, and keep working at it. If you wait until you feel 100 percent certain about your decision you're going to be waiting a long time. Sometimes you just need to take a leap.

"I'm not sure that I'm ready to give up drinking for the rest of my life." This is a big one. We've been sold the idea we must make a decision about our drinking that pertains to the rest of lives.

Here's the thing: When I started on this path, I did not make a promise to myself that I would never drink again. Even today, as I'm writing this book, that's not a promise that I've ever made to myself or to anyone else. Frankly, I don't see the utility in these promises. I think they set us up for the same black and white thinking that keeps so many people stuck in the first place.

Promises about how we are going to behave every single day for the rest of our life send us down the path of perfectionism. Either I must do something perfectly or I shouldn't bother doing it at all. I'm sure you already have examples from your own life about what happens when you set yourself to be "perfect." If you have a setback, you're not quick to jump back into the saddle. You beat yourself up. You tell yourself you failed again. You might even decide that since you've already screwed up you might as well go whole hog.

By telling myself that I wasn't making a decision for the rest of my life, it took away so much pressure at the very beginning. Today, I don't drink because I don't desire to drink, not because I've made a solemn oath never to do so again or told myself that I can't. At the same time, I also have a really clear picture of what's important to me and what I want my life to look like, and I make my decisions in accordance with those values and goals. In a strange way, taking away the threat of "I must give up drinking forever or else I'm letting myself down" actually allowed me to feel more confident.

Exercise 7: Your Complete Picture

Time Required: 1 hour

When most people decide to change their drinking, they focus on altering *how much* they drink (their aftermath problems). It makes a lot of sense. After all, your desire to change is most likely rooted in the fact that you don't like the repercussions of drinking too much. For example:

- Waking up the next morning feeling groggy, headachy, and nauseated.
- Worrying about what you said or did the previous night.
- Picking fights with friends or loved ones.
- Not remembering everything that happened or the loss of control.
- Feeling like you rely too much on alcohol to help you relax or loosen up.
- Needing alcohol to help you escape or numb your feelings.
- Disliking the pull that alcohol has over you or the worrying that it might be a problem.

Your reasons for wanting to change your drinking are specific to you, but I guarantee that you're already familiar with the downsides. I hope that the very first exercise in this book, How Does Your Drinking Help You?, started to shift your thinking by looking at your drinking from a different perspective. After all, if there weren't any upsides, you wouldn't want to drink in the first place. Here's where Exercise 7: Your Complete Picture, comes in. The goal is to identify your unique costs and *benefits* when it comes to both drinking and not drinking.

The information you list here is just that—information. What you include is neither good nor bad. There are no right or wrong answers. Try to think of your responses as data points. The more data points you have, the better you can assess where you want to go from here. Ultimately, the decisions about if and how you want to change are yours.

Once you have a complete picture of the role drinking plays in your life, you may discover that, instead of devoting all your energy to controlling how much you drink, it feels good devoting some of that energy to learning new avenues to give yourself the same benefits. You might discover that the benefits you list peak with your first glass and wane as you keep going. You may also decide that you aren't ready to take a break, which is okay too. The point of the worksheet is not to persuade you to stop, but to create a 360-degree assessment of your drinking.

The chart included here is a sample. It is filled in with the responses from one of my clients so you can see what a completed chart looks like. You'll want to fill it in with your own response (you can create one of your own or download a template here: www.rachelhart.com/book-freebie.) The top two boxes are where you list the benefits and costs associated with your drinking as it currently stands. The bottom two boxes are where you list the benefits and costs associated with stopping drinking.

I encourage you to stick to the single-page format so that you can see all the benefits and costs associated with drinking and not-drinking in one place. Some people find having it on a single sheet of paper makes it easier for them to slip it into their wallet and pull it out when they want a reminder about why they are practicing these tools. Once you finish, make sure you re-read Your Complete Picture. Do you think that it captures everything? Is there anything else you should add or include?

YOUR DRINKING RIGHT NOW	
Benefits	Costs
What do you like about drinking? What situations does it make better? What does it help you cope with? How does it help you?	*How can your drinking negatively affect your health, relationships, emotions, productivity, etc.? What concerns do you have if nothing changes?*
• Helps me relax. • Helps me socialize. • Helps me open up with people I don't know. • Feel less awkward about myself when drinking. • Helps me meet guys. • Have fun with people—breaks down barriers. • Laughing/being silly. • Quiets my inner critic. • Gets me out of my head. • Helps me stop being so fixated on myself.	• Waking up hung-over and feeling physically terrible for an entire day. • The shame I feel after a particularly bad night. • Being embarrassed about something I said or did. • Not remembering what happened. • Making connections with people that don't last. • Making risky choices around men and safety.

NOT DRINKING	
Benefits	Costs
Are there benefits from not drinking: e.g., physical/emotional health, relationships, sex, memory, money, productivity? What activities/experiences do you enjoy more without alcohol?	*What are the downsides of not having alcohol in your life? What would be less enjoyable? What situations/relationships would be more difficult?*
• I would be tons more productive. Instead of thinking about all of this I could be working to accomplish something positive. • I would have a lot more time by getting rid of the time wasted on evenings that start out as a glass of wine only to turn into hours and hours down the drain, plus the time I spend in bed hung-over. • I would have more money. So much is wasted on drinking. • I would be proud of myself. • I wouldn't wake up after a night of drinking in a funk. • I wouldn't feel like I was fooling people; like I was this put together person on the outside, and totally messed up person on the inside. • I would remember everything that happens. • I would feel less guilty about a bad night. • Hopefully my sleep would improve and be less disturbed. • Lose weight.	• Will always be on the outside. Will stick out as different. • Life will be boring • I will remain uptight and appear that way to others. • Will never be able to just have fun with my girlfriends. • Will have to wear a label and tell people something is wrong with me. • Won't be able to celebrate with people. • Can't be normal and just have a glass of wine with dinner.

What's Really Going to Motivate You?

By now you should have a complete list of the costs and benefits associated with drinking and not drinking.

I tried to make a decision about what to do about my drinking more times than I can count. It always focused on being embarrassed about something I had done or said and waking up the next day feeling regretful and hung over. I thought that just reminding myself of the consequences of drinking too much would be the solution. You've probably done the same thing. You've probably focused on all the reasons why you shouldn't drink. Maybe you've made long lists of the repercussion. All the bad things you've ever done or said. All the downsides (i.e., the aftermath problems).

The reason this doesn't work is because you're trying to use shame as a motivator for change, and shame is a terrible motivator. Shame only reminds you of all the ways you've failed, not lived up to your standards, or done something wrong. It might convince you in the short-term that you need to change your ways, but when shame is driving the process of transformation you're going to give up. Reminding yourself over and over again of the horrible hangovers and bad decisions is not going to keep you from repeating the same outcomes. The painful repercussions of over-drinking are not going to keep you in line. They just keep you focused on the past when really you should be looking toward the future.

If you're not convinced, just remember the cycle, think → feel → act. When the thought you have for wanting to change is, "When I drink, I'm an idiot," the cycle isn't working in your favor because it's not producing a feeling that makes you feel motivated to keep going even when things get tough. Not to mention when we are ashamed of ourselves, we are not only likely to run and hide but also to feel like we need a respite from ourselves. If you're practiced at using alcohol as a crutch, guess what this often leads to: drinking to feel better.

You need to find a thought that is going to motivate you to *want* to change. But as discussed all the way back in Chapter 2, there are real benefits to your drinking, otherwise you wouldn't keep doing it. Not only does the thought have to motivate you to keep going when things get tough, it has to be *stronger* than whatever thought is motivating you not to change and stay with the status quo. Figuring out a truly motivating thought all comes down to answering two questions:

- Why do you want to keep drinking?
- Why do you want to take a break?

It's a simple as that. When you start answering these questions, you'll start to have a very clear understanding if your reasons for taking a break can compete with your reasons for keeping things the same.

For years, I never looked at my decision in this light. I knew the pros and cons, and was really good at using the cons to beat myself up and try to make myself change. Sometimes it would work for a while, but usually I would slip back into my old habits. I didn't understand why my resolve kept failing. The only answer I had was that something must be wrong with me. But nothing was wrong with me. I just hadn't identified a reason to stop drinking that could stand up to my reason to keep things the same.

This is what I discovered when I started trying to answer these questions:

- **Why do you want to keep drinking?** *Because I want to fit in and be normal.*
- **Why do you want to take a break?** *Because I'm sick of the hangovers and doing things that I'm embarrassed about or regret.*

When I saw my answers head to head, I suddenly realized why I always went back to drinking. My motivation to stop drinking seemed pretty good. I truly did not like how I physically felt the next day or the embarrassment and regret that I experienced. But for me the reason to stop drinking couldn't compete with my desire to keep things the same. Wanting to fit in and be normal was my trump card. When push came to shove, it would always win, and by extension my commitment to taking a break was actually very flimsy. I would ultimately always choose being normal over being hung-over and regretful. For me, being normal was the biggest prize of all. How could I give up on that?

It seems simple, but the strength of your motivation and commitment comes down to this: Can your reason for stopping compete with your reason for keeping the status quo? If it can't, then it's going to be very hard to stick with your commitment because it won't be important enough for you. You have to be invested. You have to believe that you are getting more from stopping than you are from the status quo.

It may take you some time to figure out a reason for taking a break that can stand up to your reason for keeping things the same. Just because you don't identify one on the first try doesn't mean that you've done anything wrong or that you'll never be able to find a reason. It only means that you're going to have to keep looking. After a lot of brainstorming on my part, I finally came up with these answers:

- **Why do you want to keep drinking?** *Because I want to fit in and be normal.*
- **Why do you want to take a break?** *Because I want to be proud of who I am.*

This was what worked for me. Your reason will be unique to you and is different for all of my clients. In my case, being proud of myself not only could stand toe to toe with my desire to be normal, but it actually was more important to me. If you remember my story in Chapter 1, I talked about choosing the college I went to because I wanted to be a woman who would make a difference in the world. That had always been a strong motivation for me, and my desire to do something that would make me proud of myself was very strong.

This isn't to say that once I found this motivation I was able to let go of my desire to be normal. It was still there, and it was still something that I had to work on. I had to work on dismantling this thought and the idea that drinking and being normal went hand in hand. On the face of it, the thought, "I just want to be normal" sounds benign, but for me it was a truly negative thought that had terrible results. If being normal only came from being able to drink like everyone else, then I would always feel like I was on the outside and different. Not drinking would always feel negative to me, if I continued to associate it with being "normal." Ultimately, you need to do the work to find an answer that works for you.

Deciding on a Timeframe

Once you have your motivation, you'll want to figure out how long a period to set aside to work on these tools. Even though you are setting aside a certain number of days, be careful not to focus all your attention on reaching a number milestone. When most people focus only on counting days, their focus is squarely on using willpower—gritting their teeth and getting through one day so that they can make it to the next. There's nothing wrong with needing to grit your teeth when you start out. When this happens, go back to Exercise 5 on how to sit with an urge. You want to make sure you're practicing developing more sustainable skills than just willpower. Counting days can serve as evidence that you're capable of not drinking, but it won't help you undo negative thought patterns, get comfortable sitting with negative emotions, or learn how to observe an urge. In short, counting days helps you learn that you can not drink, but it doesn't teach you how to stop using alcohol as a crutch.

With this in mind, it is helpful to set aside a period of time when you're going to work on practicing these tools. I suggest setting aside a minimum of 30 days. Consistently working on these tools over this period will give you a fair amount of practice. You can think of it this way: it's not the number of days that you are abstaining but the length of time that you have set aside to practice the exercises. What if you're not ready to take a break? Of course, these tools are the easiest to learn and implement when you're not dealing with the repercussions of over-drinking. But progress can still be made if you decide to keep drinking. **Remember, if you do drink during your break period, all is not lost. There's no need to restart the clock or begin again from zero. Just pick yourself up and keep practicing.**

Practicing the Tools

You'll outline your plan in Exercise 8. You'll notice that three tools make up the foundation of your break period. You can practice as many tools as you want, but these three will create a solid framework as you work toward not needing to rely on alcohol as a crutch:

- Observing Your Thoughts (Exercise 2)
- Observing Your Emotions (Exercise 4)
- Observing Your Urges (Exercise 5)

As a baseline, you should practice these tools at least 100 times. I know that seems like a lot, but each tool requires only 10 minutes. Completing all three tools every day takes no more than 30 minutes total. You've spent a lot of time practicing using alcohol as a crutch, if you're going to undo this habit, you need to set aside time to practice the tools that will help you learn a new way forward. You can commit 30 minutes a day toward this goal.

Do You Have to Stop Drinking during Your Plan?

If you want to learn how to stop using alcohol as a crutch, you are going to have to practice sitting with emotions that you are used to numbing with a drink. You'll also need to practice experiencing situations where the urge to drink arises and not drink (e.g., coming home from work, socializing). Can you practice these tools even if you decide not to take a hiatus from drinking? Of course. Is your progress going to be slower? You bet.

I'm guessing this is not the news you want to hear, and I understand. You have a lot of thoughts about what it means not to drink. (Now might be a good time to go back and review Exercise 3: Identifying Your Stories About Alcohol.) Remember these stories, while they may feel true to you, are all optional. When you've thought these stories for a long time, it will take both practice and experience to start thinking differently. Let's say when you filled out Exercise 3 you came up with the following stories:

- People who don't drink are buzz-kills.
- Drinking is necessary for dating.
- Drinking makes me fun.
- Life without drinking would be boring.

Do you think it would be possible to disprove these stories if you're still drinking? Can you see how difficult it would be to disprove these stories while you continue to drink? Therein lies the benefit of taking a break. Again, you don't have to. You can still practice the tools, but your progress will be slower.

The plan outlined in Exercise 8 assumes you're taking a break. You're not deciding what you're going to do with the rest of your life. You're not swearing off ever having a champagne toast at a wedding. You're not committing to never having a beer at the ballpark. You're making a decision about what you're ready to do right now and for at least the next 30 days.

If you're not ready, that's okay too. A lot of people I talk to are interested in these concepts and want things to change, but they aren't ready to commit to taking a break from drinking. As I mentioned earlier, don't let the "right time" or feeling "ambivalent" stop you from trying something new. But if you decide not to take a break, don't let that be the reason not to practice the tools. You can practice them even if you drink—for instance by pausing to observe and describe the urge to drink *before* you pour yourself a glass.

Exercise 8: Put Your Plan on Paper

Time Required: 1 hour

These three sections will help you outline your motivation, focus, and timeframe in order to create a successful plan to take a break from drinking so that you can practice the tools and learn how to stop using alcohol as a crutch. You can practice as many tools as you like, but three exercises will be key: Observing Your Thoughts, Observing Your Emotions, and Observing Urges. These exercises make up the foundation of your work and will help build a solid foundation to unlearn your desire to drink. Download a plan template at www.rachelhart.com/book-freebie.

PART 1: Find Your Motivation

The first step is to find a thought that is truly going to motivate you to *want* to change. Start by answering the following questions:

- **Why do you want to keep drinking?**
- **Why do you want to take a break?**

Look at your answers. Do you think they're an honest reflection of where you are right now and what you really believe? Make sure you don't skip the first question, "Why do you want to keep drinking?"

Sometimes the clients I work with worry that by even acknowledging the desire to keep drinking they are going to stay stuck. Avoiding answering the question doesn't mean that you won't ever think about the benefits, especially when an urge comes up. Ignoring the benefits will only make it less likely that you're able to find a truly motivating reason to take a break.

Now it's time to assess whether your reason for wanting to take a break can stand up to your reason for wanting to keep things the same:

- **Do you feel motivated by your reason for wanting to take a break?**
- **Can your reason for wanting to take a break stand up to your reason for wanting to keep drinking?**
- **Do you think your reason for taking a break will sustain you when you're frustrated and questioning the utility of sticking with your plan?**
- **If not, brainstorm at least five possible reasons for taking a break that would be more motivating.** *Don't worry if you don't come up with a truly motivating reason on the first try. It may take some time to figure out something that motivates you. The more you brainstorm, the more likely you are to find a reason that will work for you.*

PART 2: Identify Your Focus
Remember your goal is not to stop drinking for its own sake. You're undertaking this work so that you can learn how to stop using alcohol as a crutch. Go back and review Exercise 1: How Does Drinking Help You? Based on your responses, answer the following questions:

- **What are the situations in which you want to learn how to stop using alcohol as a crutch?**

- **What are the specific emotions you want to get more comfortable with?**

These two areas will be the focus of your plan during your break.

PART 3: Set a Timeframe

Now that you have a truly motivating reason and your areas of focus, you'll need to decide how long you want to take a break and practice these tools. I suggest setting aside a minimum of 30 days, but you can also opt to set aside more time. There's no right or wrong answer when it comes to picking a number of days. Some people prefer to start small and add time as they go. Other people are motivated by bigger numbers. Ultimately, the days are only as useful as your commitment to practicing the tools.

- **How long will you commit to working on these tools?**
- **Why have you decided on this amount of time?**
- **Do you feel good about this number?**

Once you feel confident about your motivation, focus, and timeframe, you'll want to put your plan on paper along with the tools you're committed to practicing. You can download a template at www.rachelhart.com/book-freebie.

Assessing Your Progress

You've made a plan, and you're working through the exercises. But how do you know if you're making progress? Think back to the example of touch-typing from earlier in this chapter. Even if something makes sense intellectually, unlearning one habit and learning a new one takes time and consistent practice. Often, we're so focused on getting to where a new habit is completely unconscious (i.e., where it comes almost naturally without thinking about it) that we view our progress only through the lens: "Is this easy yet?"

The tools *will* get easier the longer you practice them, but focusing on ease above everything else is not particularly helpful. In fact, it can kill your motivation. Every time you run into an obstacle or an exercise feels difficult or frustrating, you can get caught up in wondering why this feels so hard. Remember, change is hard. It takes work. Don't let the difficulties you encounter be discouraging. Challenges are a sign that your brain is trying to learn something new. The worst thing you can do is tell yourself that something has gone wrong if the exercises aren't easy. Nothing has gone wrong. **If you're practicing the tools, you're doing them the right way. Practice is the key here, not perfection.**

The same is true if you walk into a situation in which you used to rely on alcohol to help make it easier and are frustrated that you feel uncomfortable without a drink in your hand. Remember that the ability to experience discomfort is part of what you are learning to do. **You are supposed to feel uncomfortable.** The ability to tolerate discomfort and not numb it with alcohol is the real goal. Do not make the mistake of thinking that the goal is to never be uncomfortable. Not only is that counter-productive, it's also impossible. Negative emotions are a part of life.

The following questions can help you look at your progress through a different lens than "Is this easy yet?" You can check in with these questions at any point during your break period. They are especially helpful at the end of a break period to help you determine whether you want to extend your break:

- Do you feel more connected to what you're thinking throughout the day and less like you're on auto-pilot?
- Are you starting to get a sense for how your thoughts create specific emotions?

- Have you noticed the think → feel → act cycle in action?
- Have you discovered that your thoughts are optional?
- Have you practiced new thoughts and made headway with them?
- Are you finding alternate ways of thinking about a single situation?
- Have you noticed any thoughts that seem to be on repeat? (Often people discover that there are certain thoughts that crop up again and again throughout the day.)
- Do you have a new understanding of how emotions feel in your body?
- Are you able to describe with precision the way different emotions feel?
- Have you found that your tolerance for certain emotions has grown?
- Are you able to describe what an urge feels like in your body?
- Have you watched an urge arise, peak, and pass?
- Have you noticed your urges in other parts of your life and brought mindfulness to them?
- Do you feel like you can tolerate your urges at least sometimes?
- Have you brought more attention to unconscious habits like walking or driving?
- Do you have an understanding of the thoughts that fuel your desire to drink?
- Have you started to question some of your stories about alcohol?

These questions should help you turn your attention away from whether this process is "easy" and focus on the different areas of progress.

But what about what happens when you reach the end of the time period that you set aside? How do you decide about where to go from there? The most important thing is not to rush into anything. If you feel yourself rushing to get to day 31 so that you can start drinking, you know that you still have work to do. Wanting to move quickly and get back to drinking can mean that you're relying too much on willpower and may need more practice with the tools.

Remember, the goal is not to stop drinking, the goal is to stop using alcohol as a crutch for the parts of your life where you experience discomfort. Go back to Exercise 1: How Does Drinking Help You? and review your answers to the following questions:

- What situations does alcohol improve or make easier?
- List any specific emotions alcohol helps with.

You want to consider the progress you've made in these two areas. If you feel like you have more work to do, keep going. At some point, you want to be capable of dealing with the situations and emotions on your own.

Finally, Exercise 7: Your Complete Picture, gave you a sense of what you thought the benefits of not drinking would be. Now that you have a break period under your belt, go back and answer the questions from Exercise 7 again. See if you can find any new benefits to list:

- What are the benefits from not drinking: e.g., physical/emotional health, relationships, sex, memory, money, productivity?
- What activities/experiences do you enjoy more without alcohol?

This information together with your assessment of where you are on using alcohol as a crutch and your progress on the tools should help you decide whether you want to continue working on learning how to stop using alcohol as a crutch.

7 Overcoming Common Obstacles

Handling Peoples' Questions

O nce I made a decision to take a break, I was suddenly really worried about what other people would think. Trying to figure out how to stop using alcohol as a crutch was one thing. Talking about this decision was another. At times, fielding people's questions about why I wasn't drinking seemed more difficult than actually not drinking. I hated telling people I didn't drink. I hated answering their questions about why I couldn't just moderate. I hated having to explain myself.

Why? For starters, I didn't have great answers. I knew that moderating sometimes worked and sometimes didn't, and I had no idea why. I knew that I used alcohol as a crutch, but I believed it was a problem unique to me. But more than anything, it took me a long time to shake my own acceptance of the predominate narratives about people who struggle with alcohol. I saw my struggle as something that was wrong with me.

I concocted stories about needing to wake up early or that I wasn't drinking as part of a cleanse or a diet. I told people I wasn't feeling well or that I was taking antibiotics. My excuses rarely worked. People told me that they too had to wake up early, and I should join in. They offered up a vodka and soda as a low-calorie option or explained that red wine was okay in moderation on cleanse. Once I even got into a debate with a bunch of people who tried to convince me it was safe to mix antibiotics and alcohol—they did it all the time.

All of this made me want to shut myself away in my apartment and never come out. But stopping all human interaction wasn't sustainable. I wanted to see my friends. I wanted to go to parties. I wanted to hang out with coworkers after work and not have it be a big deal. I wanted to live my life, which meant coming up with an answer to the question, "How come you're not drinking?" Finding the right response felt like I was preparing for cross-examination. I wanted to be prepared for every potential follow up question. I thought I had to have really good reasons to prove that not drinking and being normal could go together.

People would ask why I wasn't drinking and I would tell them, "I just decided to stop." Nine times out of ten they came back with a million follow up questions. It seemed people were always dying to know more. I walked away feeling like I had been interrogated. Why wouldn't people just leave me alone?

Here's what I finally realized. The more I thought that the fact that I didn't drink was a big deal, the more the energy behind my answer felt like some deep, dark secret. Unsurprisingly, when people encountered this energy from me, they wanted to dig deeper. My body language, my tone of voice, everything said, "I had something to hide" and when people come face to face with a secret they become intrigued and want to know more. When I thought my not drinking was a big deal, it became a big deal. When I was terrified that not drinking meant something unredeemable about me, it came through in the energy behind my words. I didn't deliver them in a self-assured, who-cares kind of way because I didn't believe my answer was a who-cares kind of thing. I thought it meant something about me. I thought not drinking was a big deal.

Here's where the think → feel → act cycle comes into play. Not drinking was the fact. My answer to why I was drinking, in other words, what I thought about that fact, determined how I felt (my emotion), and how I delivered my response (how I acted). Here's how the cycle looked when I first started out and what it looks like now:

Someone asks me why I don't drink (when I first started).

- **Think**: "If I tell them I quit they're going to think that something is wrong with me" →
- **Feel**: embarrassed →
- **Act**: Clam up and deliver my response in a halting, unnatural way.

Someone asks me why I don't drink (now).

- **Think**: "Not drinking has absolutely no bearing on who I am as a person" →
- **Feel**: secure →
- **Act**: Tell them I don't drink without making a big deal about it.

It all comes down to what you make it mean that you aren't drinking. I was choosing to think that it was a sign that something was wrong with me rather than an insignificant detail among the hundreds, if not thousands, of details about who I was as a person. I didn't move from

"Something is wrong with me" to "It's not a big deal" overnight. But shifting your perspective is entirely possible.

If you feel uncomfortable answering peoples' questions, it's because you're uncomfortable with what you think your answer means about you. The thing is, you get to decide. Remember it's less about having the perfect response and more about what you decide your answer means about you.

Dealing with Friends and Loved Ones

I'll be honest with you, not everyone thought my not drinking was a great idea. Some of my friends were really proud of me, others wanted to know how long this was going to last and pushed me to make an exception (just this once). There were boyfriends who were supportive, and boyfriends who thought that I should be able to moderate. There were first dates that didn't notice, and first dates that went south as soon as it became clear I would not be splitting a bottle of wine over dinner.

In the beginning, I interpreted anything even remotely questioning as unsupportive. I wanted everyone to be 100 percent on board, and not everyone was. Here's what I learned: wanting the entire world to support my decision not to drink was not only unrealistic, it pointed to a deeper issue. The truth was I had doubts. Was stopping the right decision? Did it mean something about me? Could I even see this through?

I didn't realize it at the time, but wanting the entire world to support my decision was my way of protecting myself. I wanted everyone's unwavering support so I could avoid the hard work of facing my doubts. When it comes to our closest relationships, we all have expectations for other people's behavior. The important thing is not to confuse getting your expectations met with determining how you feel. Here's what I mean: I want to be treated with kindness, love, compassion, and fairness in my relationships. That said, I know my happiness is not dependent on others' treating me this way. Frankly, I'm not going to always get what I want.

Remember the think → feel → act cycle. Your feelings aren't created by another person's actions; they're created by the thoughts you have about their actions. When someone pesters you to make an exception just this once, tells you that you're no fun since you stopped drinking, or says that you're ruining dinner because they don't want to drink alone, you have to once again ask yourself, what are you making the responses mean?

If you find yourself thinking, "He shouldn't be doing this," it's a sign that you need to pay attention to your thoughts. How do you start doing this? When you find yourself upset or frustrated by someone's actions, the easiest thing to do is try to imagine his or her think → feel → act cycle and how it is working at that moment. After all, a person's actions are driven by how she feels and what she is thinking—not by what you are doing. An easy way to shift your focus is to ask yourself what the other person must be thinking or feeling in order to act this way. You don't need to excuse his or her behavior or pretend that you aren't hurt. All you need to do is shift your focus from what you think the other's actions mean about you, to what it means about that person.

I Screwed Up. Now What?

This is the sort of response I get from most clients when they have a set back: *"I was doing so well and then I had a huge setback. I feel like I've lost all the hard work I did to deal with my urges and not use alcohol as a crutch. I feel defeated. I can't believe I was so stupid."* They start going into a shame spiral. All the work and practice is out the window and the only thing they can see is how they failed. Let's pretend that you act on the urge to drink. You have one of two options.

- You can focus on how you screwed up and use it as proof that you'll never be able to figure this out, or
- You can accept that every setback is an opportunity for growth. A chance to go a little bit deeper inside what is driving the habit and figure out where the roadblock was and why you stumbled.

Most of us do the former rather than the latter. We get tunnel vision and focus on everything we think the mistake means instead of looking at it as a chance for growth. Part of this mentality goes back to the focus on counting days. The idea that if you have a setback you have to go back to zero and start over again. This never made any sense to me. You didn't lose all the time and energy that you put into your plan up until that point. All your effort hasn't been erased or undone. Think of it this way: what would you do if you fell while you were walking across a bridge? Would you walk all the way back to the beginning and start again? Not a chance. You would get up from where you fell and keep walking across.

I Feel Crappy All the Time

If you've used alcohol to cover up negative emotions, then it shouldn't be a surprise that taking a break isn't initially going to feel great. Suddenly, you're not going to have alcohol to dull your negative emotions. You may enjoy not having to deal with hangovers or waking up the next day feeling regretful about what happened the night before, but you'll also have to deal with the discomfort of not having a quick and easy way to cover up how you feel.

Here's the good news: You now have the tools to handle this. You understand the think → feel → act cycle, so you know that if you're feeling crappy it's not because a negative emotion just appeared out of thin air. You are thinking a thought that created it. This is great news. It may not feel this way at first, but remember if you can practice your thinking then you can practice letting go of whatever thought is causing you to feel a negative emotion.

The best thing to do is to go back to Exercise 2 and set aside some time to empty your thoughts on a piece of paper so that you can look at them and figure out which ones are causing you to feel the negative emotion. You can also go back to Exercise 4 and work on observing the negative emotion and ask yourself what about the physical manifestations of the emotions is so intolerable. If you ever want to run away or cover up an emotion, it's because you think that you can't handle it. Remember, once you start paying attention to the physical changes in your body, you begin to realize that you can handle whatever emotion comes your way.

Numbing vs. Comforting

It's not uncommon when you take a break from alcohol to discover that you've found something new to replace distracting and numbing yourself from how you're feeling. This is totally normal. Your brain has a well-worn pathway of dealing with negation emotions by trying to cover them up.

All the tools that you've learned in this book will help you with anything you use to numb how you're feeling. But first you need to determine whether you're numbing yourself or comforting. This is such an important question for everyone to understand because almost everything you can comfort yourself with—food, money, exercise, TV, Facebook, sleep—you can also use to numb yourself.

There's nothing wrong with needing a break or wanting to soothe yourself. Being able to tend to yourself is an important skill. The thing is, few of us are ever taught how to care for ourselves or how to tell if we are comforting ourselves or numbing something we don't want to feel. The point is not to focus on the substance or activity but to examine how you feel during and after.

- **Numbing feels fast and insatiable.** There's always an urge for more; you feel like you can't pull yourself away or get enough. While the effect lasts, you may feel numbed, dulled, zoned out, or as if you have escaped reality. Afterwards, you rarely feel good. More likely, you feel depleted. You might even feel ashamed. Many women find this to be true with drinking, but also with the myriad other ways that they try to dull the things they don't want to feel.

- **Comfort feels steady and time-bound.** You're not pushing yourself to keep going; you're setting aside time thoughtfully and deliberately. You remain conscious and aware throughout. Afterwards, you feel replenished and in a better frame of mind to tackle something that you know is going to be hard. You feel more ready to face whatever was going on.

Going back to Chapter 1, it's the difference between problem-solving and problem-stalling. Comforting gets you ready for problem-solving. It's the breather you need so you can start to resolve whatever isn't working. Numbing is problem-stalling. It's turning to the same activity over and over again so you don't have to face what you don't want to feel. Not only that, but numbing usually creates its own set of new problems. Now you have to deal with the negative repercussions of over-drinking, over-eating, over-spending, or over-watching.

Encountering obstacles during your journey is normal. In fact, I would argue that experiencing all of the obstacles outlined in this chapter only makes you more resilient and better able to cope with whatever comes your way. Trying to structure everything so you never have to answer questions or face disapproval from others is a lot like attempting to live in a bubble.

Setbacks are part of the process. You don't need to freak out when they happen. You don't have to wonder if all your work was for naught.

The important thing is to decide to keep plugging away even in the face of obstacles. You taught yourself to use alcohol as a crutch, and now you have to teach yourself a new way forward.

8   How to Feel Better

U ltimately, you want to do more than to stop using alcohol as a crutch. You also want to feel better more often. The think → feel → act cycle will help you challenge negative thought patterns and generate better emotions.

Challenging Negative Thought Patterns

When it comes to feeling better, you need to do more than just observe your thoughts. You need to actually change negative thought patterns.

Social anxiety was a huge issue for me. When I started doing this work, I noticed that when I was in an unfamiliar social situation I kept thinking the same thought over and over again: "I don't fit in here." This made me feel profoundly awkward and uncomfortable. I would fixate on everything that was wrong with me: My outfit was ugly. I hated the way I looked. All the other women had something that I didn't. The more awkward and uncomfortable I felt, the more I clammed up.

I didn't participate. I didn't smile. My body was tense and closed off. Everything about me read, "Don't talk to me." And sure enough, in that state, I didn't fit in. The only way I knew how to relieve this feeling was by having a drink.

My solution was to try and "fix" myself. I thought if I could master how I looked on the outside I could feel better on the inside. You know now, that's not how the think → feel → act cycle works. By paying attention to what I was thinking, how those thoughts made me feel, and when I felt that way, how I acted, suddenly I had a different place to focus my attention. It wasn't a matter of walking into a party and saying to myself over and over, "I fit in, I fit in" because I never would have believed those words. I had to find a new, believable thought that I could practice thinking instead of what was normally on repeat in my head: I don't fit in.

What actually started to change things for me was practicing thinking, "I'm sure there is someone else here who feels just as out of place as I do." It seems like such a small change, but it gave me a little bit of relief. It made me feel less alone. I could relax the tiniest bit. Breathe a little better. It was just enough space to feel like I could get through the first 30 minutes of a party (which to me were always the worst) without needing to drink.

Small shifts in your thinking can have a big change. Take for example shame versus guilt. Clearly, neither is a positive emotion. But most people recognize that shame, for some reason, feels much worse. Why is that? You can think of it as the difference between the thought, "I am bad" and "I did something bad." These thoughts are almost identical, yet they produce totally different feelings. "I am bad" produces shame: it has to do with who you are as a person—something that is fundamental to your very being. Whereas, "I did something bad" creates guilt. It still doesn't feel good, but it's nowhere as suffocating as the feeling of shame because "I did something bad" focuses on the behavior rather than the person. Sometimes just moving myself from shame to guilt by changing my thoughts feels a hundred times better.

You are the only person that is capable of changing your thoughts. Instinctively you already know this. People can tell you you're smart, beautiful, funny, they can tell you to cut yourself slack or be kinder to yourself, but if you don't believe these things yourself, their words will never stick. You have to find a way to start to believe something different for yourself. The skill of seeing how your thoughts affect you and practicing new, better-feeling thoughts is the basis of this work.

Exercise 2: Observing Your Thoughts, should give you good insight into what you're thinking on a regular basis. Once you have that insight, you want to see if the thoughts you think are serving you. Take a look and see if any of the following categories apply to your thoughts.

- **Notice your judgments.** Instead of thinking "I made a mistake," we think, "I made a *stupid* mistake" or we think "This feeling is *unbearable*" rather than "I'm feeling sad." "My body is *disgusting*" instead of plainly acknowledging, "This is my body." Judgments may feel true, but they're always optional.

- **Look for all-or-nothing statements.** Have you set up parameters that only focus on the negative and ignore the neutral or positive? "I *completely* neglect my body." "He *always* gives me a hard time." "I *never* get things right." "*No one* likes me." "This is *impossible*." Even if you feel a statement is 99.9% true, acknowledging the .01% can start to provide relief. For example, "I sometimes take care of my body." "He is giving me a hard time right now." "I make mistakes sometimes." "There are people in my life who love me." "This is difficult but not impossible."

- **Are you fighting what is?** Instead of acknowledging the reality of the situation, we fixate on how we wish things were. "I'm trying to change my drinking" becomes "Why me?" or "It isn't fair that this is a problem that I have to deal with." When we acknowledge how things actually are, we can turn our attention to problem solving, rather than staying stuck in a thought pattern that focuses on wanting something to be different than it is.

- **Using the word "should" and deciding how things ought to be.** The word should feels neutral, but it often produces a negative feeling. "Should" fuels the belief that if only we could control how things happened and how people behaved then we could finally feel better. To see how this works, whenever you notice the should, ask yourself "What's the unspoken "why" that I've attached to it? For example: "She shouldn't talk to me that way" (Why? Because then I wouldn't be angry.) "He shouldn't be so impatient in line." (Why? Because it's rude, and rude people annoy me.) "I should lose 10 lbs." (Why? Because then I could finally feel good about myself.) "I should have this figured out by now. (Why? Because then I wouldn't be stressed out.). Try restating your thought without using "should."

- **Do your thoughts contain unreasonable standards?** Has your thinking set up a framework where it's not okay for you to fail, make mistakes, or be anything less than perfect? High standards can be great—they can push us to stretch beyond our limits and accomplish wonderful things. But not if they don't take into account that we are human and we will fail, backslide, and make mistakes. They are used as a weapon against ourselves rather than as a means for betterment. We need standards that give us space to be complicated, messy, and flawed.

Once you've identified certain thoughts that aren't serving you, the next step is to brainstorm new, better-feeling thoughts and give them a spin. It's important to remember that coming up with new, better-feeling thoughts is *not* the same as positive thinking. You can choose better-feeling thoughts without turning into a Pollyanna. You don't need to anticipate the best possible outcome or see only the good in people. All you need to do is find a new thought that feels both believable and slightly better. If the thought isn't believable, then no matter how many times you repeat it, it's not going to change how you feel.

For example, if you consistently tell yourself "People who don't drink are boring," then switching to "People who don't drink are fun" is going to fall flat. It's just not possible for your brain to go from disdain to admiration overnight. (That's why people often say that repeating affirmations feels fake.) It's best to go from a negative thought to a neutral one (e.g., from "People who don't drink are boring" to "Some people don't drink"). When you think about going to a party and not drinking and catch yourself thinking "People who don't drink are boring," you can replace it with "Some people don't drink."

Don't worry. You're not going to be stuck with neutral thought forever, but you have to go about creating new thought patterns gradually. You'll know when you feel ready to try out a new, more positive thought (e.g., from "Some people don't drink" to "I can be fun and not drink"). Think of it as climbing the steps on a staircase. Pick one or two thoughts you want to work on and start brainstorming as many new, believable possibilities as you can. You'll know when you hit on something that feels good to you. Here are some examples to get you started:

Negative Thoughts	Neutral Thoughts
I made a stupid mistake.	I made a mistake.
This feeling is horrible.	I am feeling/I can tolerate [insert emotion].
My body is disgusting.	This is my body.
I completely neglect my body.	I can care for my body.

He always gives me a hard time.	This is just John being John.
I never get things right.	Sometimes I make mistakes.
No one likes me.	Some people like me.
This is impossible.	This is hard, but I'm figuring it out.
I don't want to be injured.	I have a broken arm.
I'm never going to feel better.	I can get through today.
She shouldn't talk to me that way.	I wonder what's making her act this way?
He shouldn't be so impatient.	Everyone gets impatient sometimes.
I should lose 10lbs.	I weigh 150lbs.
I should've figured this out already.	I can see this through/It's okay if it takes time.

If you're struggling to come up with believable, neutral thoughts, here are some tips:

- **What would you say to a friend or a loved one who told you she was thinking this negative thought?** It's often easier to think about how we would assess a situation if a friend or loved one was in our position.
- **If you are struggling with a thought about someone's behavior, see if you are able to see things from his or her perspective.** What might you think if you were in the other person's shoes? Sometimes, simply being curious about the other person's motivations and using a question as a replacement thought is enough (e.g., "I wonder what he is thinking that is making him act that way?"). At the very least, curiosity feels better than annoyed, angry, impatient, or unworthy.

Once you have a thought that you want to try out, you have to start incorporating it into your life. You'll need a two-pronged approach:

- **Repetition**: Learning a new thought is like learning a new song. It's unlikely that you'll have it memorized after listening to it once. You have to put the thought on repeat. Place a sticky note where you can see it every day. Practice it silently while you brush your teeth. Set a reminder on your phone. Write it on a piece of paper and carry it in your pocket. Write the thought over and over again until you fill up an entire sheet of paper. Do whatever works for you to learn the new thought and make it a habit.
- **Replacement**: Once you've memorized the new thought, you can start to substitute it whenever the old thought appears. Remember, this isn't about getting it perfect; it's about building a habit. Every time you correct yourself and use your new thought, you are strengthening the new pathways in your brain that you need to solidify this habit.

Generating Better Emotions

Until now, the focus of this work has been on unraveling the habit of using alcohol as a crutch. Much of that work is focused on identifying the different components of the think → feel → act cycle in order to bring your habit to your consciousness and start to change it. You are working backwards with the think → feel → act cycle to understand why you feel and act the way you do. But you can also use the think → feel → act cycle forward and create how you want to feel.

Figuring this out was life-changing. I spent so many years fending off bad feelings and hoping that I would magically start feeling better. Now I actually have a framework to make that happen. Use your answers from Exercise 7: Your Complete Picture, to begin the work of generating better emotions. Start by answering the following questions. (The answers listed here are samples.)

What do you like about drinking? What situations does it make better? What does it help you cope with? How does it help you?

- *Helps me relax.*
- *Helps me to socialize.*
- *Helps me open up with people I don't know.*
- *Feel less awkward about myself when drinking.*
- *Helps me meet guys.*
- *Have fun with people—breaks down barriers.*
- *Laughing/being silly.*
- *Quiets my inner critic.*
- *Gets me out of my head.*
- *Helps me stop being so fixated on myself.*

Looking at the benefits above, what negative emotions do you think drinking help you cope with? *Stress, Awkwardness, Insecurity*

Which emotion would you like to tackle first? *Awkwardness*

When do you most often feel this emotion? *When I meet new people.*

What emotions would you like to feel instead? *Comfortable.*

Brainstorm at least 10 thoughts that could think in this situation that would generate the emotion you would like to feel instead.

- We're all in the same boat, trying to make a good first impression.
- I give people permission not to like me.
- All people worry about what other people think of them.
- I am going to approach this person with curiosity rather than apprehension.

- Someone's opinion of me has everything to do with that person.
- When I tense up I come across as tense.
- The opinion that matters the most is my own.
- If I start to feel awkward it's okay, I don't have to resist it.
- I can handle feeling awkward.
- I got this.

Select one new thought from the list that you brainstormed. Pick one that seems the most believable to you. (Don't worry about picking the "right" thought this is just a chance for you to take it on a test run.) Practice thinking this new thought before you go into the specific situation (You may want to write it down and keep it on a post-it note).

Working through these questions and finding new thoughts to practice is how you generate better feelings. This is the work that most of my clients love. Instead of just figuring out how to handle their negative thoughts and emotions, they can use the think → feel → act cycle to create positive emotions. Ultimately you can use the cycle backwards and forwards to help you understand why you feel the way you do, and create how you want to feel.

Conclusion

Why can't I drink like everyone else? This question plagued me for years and eats away at my clients. You've pondered this question too. It's why you picked up this book in the first place. During my struggle, I came up with all sorts of explanations. I couldn't drink like everyone else because "I was missing an off-switch." I couldn't drink like everyone else because "Something was wrong with me." I couldn't drink like everyone else because "I was weak-willed." I couldn't drink like everyone else because "I was broken."

I hope by now you've noticed the downside of these answers. If you plug any of these thoughts into the think → feel → act cycle you'll quickly see the negative emotions that they produce. These thoughts kept me stuck. They made me feel embarrassed, ashamed, and hopeless. When I felt this way I wanted to run and hide and ignore the problem. I had the perfect solution: have a drink and dull the pain. Repeating this question over and over in my head touched off a vicious cycle that I didn't understand.

If alcohol has become a crutch for you, it's because you unconsciously taught your brain you needed it to feel better or to get through certain situations. You practiced using alcohol over and over again to have fun, relax, loosen up, numb sadness, give you energy, help you fall asleep, alleviate boredom—the list goes on. Your brain learned that having a drink was the best way to get rid of the discomfort.

Teaching yourself this habit has absolutely no bearing on who you are as a person. There's nothing wrong with you, there's nothing wrong with your character, and there's nothing wrong with your brain. Every brain is meant to run on habits, but no one ever told you how habits work or the role of the think → feel → act cycle. When you don't understand what's fueling your desire, it's difficult to unwind it. Without this information most people are left groping in the dark, unsure of how to change what isn't working. When your attempts hit roadblocks, it's tempting to make it mean that you're just not trying hard enough or, worse still, you won't ever figure this out.

When I started this journey, all I wanted was to stop using alcohol as a crutch. I had no idea what was waiting for me on the other side. Back then, my moods were all over the place. I couldn't tolerate feeling uncomfortable, and I spent an inordinate amount of energy trying to "fix" myself so that I could be happy. When my efforts to feel better didn't work, I poured myself a drink, which unleashed a whole new round of problems.

Practicing these tools took effort. It was challenging. I had more setbacks and obstacles than I can count. Slowly something new started to emerge. It wasn't just the insight into how my habits work or a new understanding of why change was difficult. It was the realization of just how much power I had in my own life to feel better from the inside out instead of from the outside in. I learned that I could tolerate any emotion. I didn't need to numb, dull or distract myself. The more confident I became in my ability to navigate whatever came my way, the more I grew in all areas of my life. I could survive failure. I could withstand fear. I could come back from disappointment and shame.

All the hang-ups that plagued me for years started to lose their grip. Using these tools my merciless self-critic started to recede. The confidence I never had in social situations started to blossom. The perfectionist who was terrified of making mistakes started to put herself out there. I didn't need to be perfect. I didn't need to insulate myself from ever making a mistake. I could take risks, fall down, and get back up. Best of all, the nagging question, "Why can't I drink like everyone else?" started to lose its sting. I started to understand the folly in this question. How misleading it was to set up a world in which no one but me struggled.

Everyone turns to different ways of coping in order to change how they feel. There is nothing more universal in the human condition than the desire to be happy. Look around. Everywhere you turn, you'll see people searching for ways to feel better. I spent a very long time thinking that I had found the answer at the bottom of the glass. Down there I could finally feel confident, attractive and without a care. The problem was that all these feelings were fleeting. Each time I turned to a drink to feel this way, I missed out on the opportunity to learn how to generate these feelings on my own.

This is what the tools outlined in this book did for me, and what they can do for you. They opened my eyes to a different way of seeing the world. They radically transformed my relationship with myself. More than anything else, they helped me discover how to be the best version of me. I know that with practice and commitment these tools can do the same for you.

Good luck!

Acknowledgements

In the early months of my journey to learn how to stop using alcohol as a crutch, I sketched out the first outline of this book. I wasn't yet a life coach and was still trying to find my way, but for the first time I was hopeful about my future. I saw a new way forward and was excited about the tools I was learning. I was also tremendously frustrated that it had taken me over a decade to come across a positive way of understanding my struggle. This book and my work as a life coach were born out of this frustration.

So many people have helped me along the way. First and foremost my wonderful husband Tim. I couldn't ask for a better partner to have by my side. I would be remiss not to mention the following people: my parents Tom and Daria Hart and my sister Rebecca Holder and sister-in-law Molly Holder, Katie Berroth, Jonathan Birchall, Marta Brummell, Brooke Castillo, Megan Evans, Ashley Gartland, Caryn Gillen, Edward Gorecki, Stephen Grimes, Lauren Hibbert, Cynthia Kane, Eleanor Kelly,

Lorraine Kenny, Sebastian Krueger, Angela Lauria, Kara Loewentheil, Tatyana Margolin, Heather McLain, Julia Otis, Briana Paskin, Ray Robbennolt, Howard Schissler, Laura Silber, Paul Silva, Sharon Slowik, Amina Swanepoel, Katie Sweetman, Bo Tan, Radha Tilton, Susie Tofte, and everyone I met at SMART Recovery meetings on Manhattan's Upper East Side.

To the Morgan James Publishing team: Special thanks to David Hancock, CEO & Founder for believing in me and my message. To my Author Relations Manager, Margo Toulouse, thanks for making the process seamless and easy. Many more thanks to everyone else, but especially Jim Howard, Bethany Marshall, and Nickcole Watkins.

About the Author

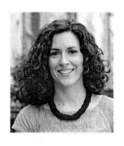 Rachel Hart is a certified life coach working in San Francisco. Her coaching focuses on the myriad ways that women disconnect from their bodies, including through alcohol. For over a decade, she worked in human rights helping activists fighting for a more just, equitable world harness their stories to create real change. Read more at her website: www.rachelhart.com.

Thank You

Thanks for reading *Why Can't I Drink Like Everyone Else?* I hope this book has given you a new framework to understand why you drink the way you do and the tools to help you change. The fact that you've gotten this far tells me you're ready to stop using alcohol as a crutch. To help you on your journey, I've put together a free template to make sure you have a rock solid plan.

Visit my website to download your free template that will keep you on track as you learn how to stop using alcohol as a crutch: <u>www.rachelhart.com/book-freebie</u>**.**

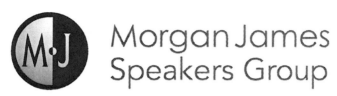

Morgan James
Speakers Group

🡕 www.TheMorganJamesSpeakersGroup.com

We connect Morgan James published
authors with live and online events
and audiences whom will benefit
from their expertise.

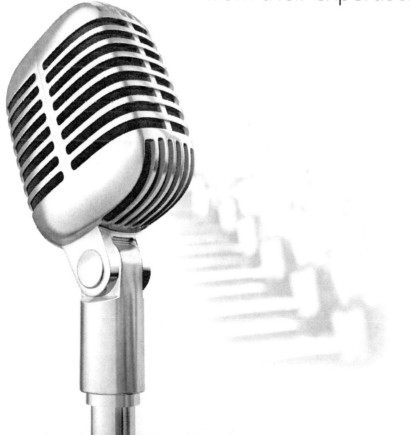

 Morgan James makes all of our titles available
through the Library for All Charity Organization.

www.LibraryForAll.org